THE PHYSIOLOGY OF
CONSCIOUSNESS

THE PHYSIOLOGY OF CONSCIOUSNESS

How Maharishi's Vedic Physiology
and Its Practical Application,
Maharishi Ayur-Ved, Can Solve the
Problems of Individual and
Collective Health and Raise Life
to a New Level of Fulfillment

ROBERT KEITH WALLACE, PH.D.

INTRODUCTION BY

John S. Hagelin, Ph.D.

Director of the Institute of Science,
Technology and Public Policy
Maharishi International University

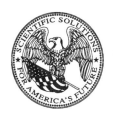

A JOINT PUBLICATION OF THE
**INSTITUTE OF SCIENCE,
TECHNOLOGY AND PUBLIC POLICY**
AND
**MAHARISHI INTERNATIONAL
UNIVERSITY PRESS**

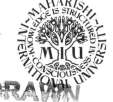

3/04

Maharishi International University Press
Fairfield, Iowa 52557 USA

Library of Congress Cataloguing-in-Publication Data

Wallace, Robert Keith, 1945–
    The physiology of consciousness / Robert Keith Wallace ;
    introduction by John S. Hagelin.
xvi, 311 p.   cm. : ; / / .
    "How Maharishi's Vedic Physiology and its practical application, Maharishi
Ayur-Ved, can solve the problems of individual and collective health and raise life
to a new level of fulfillment."
    Includes bibliographical references.
    ISBN 0-923569-02-2
    1. Medicine, Ayurvedic. 2. Consciousness. 3. Human physiology.
I. Title.
R605.W35   1993
615.5'3—dc20

The newspaper report by Jon Levy on pages 162–163 first appeared in the December 7, 1978
issue of the *Ithaca Journal*. It is reprinted here with the permission of the author.

The news report by Alex Van Oss about the "Yogic Flying Competition by Meditators" on
pages 169–171 was originally broadcast on National Public Radio's "All Things Considered" on
July 11, 1986, and is used with the permission of National Public Radio. Any unauthorized
duplication is prohibited. © copyright National Public Radio® 1986.

TO MAHARISHI MAHESH YOGI

whose unbounded compassion for humanity and

profound knowledge of the most fundamental value

of natural law is inspiring the people of all nations

to rise to perfection and create Heaven on Earth.

CONTENTS

PART 2
THE PHYSIOLOGY OF MATTER

PART 4

THE PHYSIOLOGY
OF THE UNIVERSE

ACKNOWLEDGEMENTS

I WOULD LIKE TO PARTICULARLY ACKNOWLEDGE SUSAN SHATKIN for her extraordinary achievement in editing. She went far beyond the normal boundaries of editing and made substantial scholarly and creative contributions. The depth of research, precise logic, and the heartfelt care she has given to the expression of Maharishi's Vedic Science have added immeasurably to this book.

My gratitude to Huntley Dent, Dr. Geoffrey Wells, Dr. Karen Blasdell, Phil Tomlinson, Bob Miller, Colette Guay, and Toni Alazraki for their contributions, to Shepley Hansen for the cover design, and Michael Davis and Dan Horsburgh for their expert and timely help in the book's production.

I am very grateful for the profound guidance of Dr. Bevan Morris, President of Maharishi International University, throughout this entire project.

I thank my wife Samantha for her devoted support, unfailing patience, and wisdom.

INTRODUCTION

John S. Hagelin, Ph.D.

Director of the Institute of Science,

Technology and Public Policy

Maharishi International University

I

F AMERICA IS TO CONTINUE AS A POWERFUL, POSITIVE INFLUENCE in the world, Americans must be strong and balanced in body and mind. Yet an overwhelming number of Americans suffer from poor health. Over 50 million have high blood pressure, 7 million are afflicted with heart disease, and 33 million suffer from chronic disabling conditions. Despite the billions of dollars spent on research and treatment of cancer, it is still the second leading cause of disease: 1.3 million new cases of cancer will be detected this year. As many as 76,000 will die of AIDS, almost 400,000 will die of smoking-related diseases, and 18 million will experience alcohol-related health problems.

In 1992, health care costs in the U.S. exceeded $800 billion. This vast expenditure is escalating by 15%–20% per year, while the quality of our national health is actually declining in many aspects. The high cost of health care is dramatically escalating the cost of health insurance. As a result, at least 35% of U.S. citizens are inadequately covered or have no medical insurance.

The average Fortune 1000 company spends $53 million per year on health costs, or 39% of its net profits. With the projected rise of health care costs, many of these companies will be unable to survive by the end of the decade.

This runaway growth in medical expenditures is known as the "health care crisis." It is not fundamentally a crisis of health-care delivery, of management, or of medical tort laws; the origin of this crisis is *poor health*. A new approach to *creating health* in the nation is vitally needed.

Current medical practice has no effective prevention strategy, doing little to strengthen the immune system or eliminate imbalances that are the underlying cause of disease. Indeed, it can be argued that modern medicine is responsible for a large proportion of the disease that afflicts our society. For example, iatrogenic disease, disorders caused as a result of medical treatment, has been shown in several studies to account for about one-third of health problems seen in hospitals. Thus the health care crisis is far more fundamental than delivery of existing health care; it is a problem of the very world view upon which modern medicine is based.

The limitations of modern medicine are rooted in the materialistic, reductionistic viewpoint of nineteenth-century science. Although these ideas were revolutionary in their time, we must now adopt a more modern world view based on the more complete scientific understanding of nature provided by quantum mechanics and unified quantum field theories. These theories identify a single, universal field of intelligence at the basis of mind and matter—a single field which underlies and gives rise to all forms and phenomena in the universe. They replace the partial and fragmented understanding of isolated laws of nature provided by classical physics with a comprehensive and holistic understanding which highlights the fundamentally unified structure of natural law.

It is of paramount importance that twentieth-century medicine become based on twentieth-century science. Through its reliance on classical concepts, current medical practice, despite its successes, is conceptually primitive, and at times barbaric in its approach to the physiology. Its fragmented, disease-oriented approach to the body causes side effects, creates physiological imbalance, and sows the seeds for future disease. To be truly effective, medicine must take advantage of the more comprehensive, up-to-date, and holistic understanding of nature provided by twentieth-century science. It is time for a new medical paradigm based on the unified field.

It is extremely interesting that this new medical paradigm, which is brilliantly described by Dr. Robert Keith Wallace in this book, has historical roots in the most ancient tradition of knowledge in the world—

the Vedic tradition of India. Maharishi Mahesh Yogi, the founder of Transcendental Meditation, has worked with modern scientists and scholars of the Vedic tradition to bring to light from the Vedic litera-ture a wealth of knowledge and practical technologies based on the most profound and comprehensive understanding of natural law. The result of this work, known as Maharishi's Vedic Science and Tech-nology, has immense practical significance for the health and life of every individual and every society.

The Physiology of Consciousness is about the rediscovery of this knowl-edge and Dr. Wallace's contribution to its powerful and timely resur-gence. Over the last twenty years, Dr. Wallace has had the rare privi-lege of working closely with Maharishi in restoring and interpreting the ancient wisdom of the Ved in the contemporary language of mod-ern medicine. Dr. Wallace is world-renowned for his pioneering research in the physiology of Transcendental Meditation and higher states of consciousness. His groundbreaking studies in the early 1970s have had enormous impact on the fields of psychophysiology and behavioral medicine. They have stimulated literally hundreds of scien-tific publications on the physiology, biochemistry, psychology, and soci-ological effects of higher states of consciousness.

In this book, Dr. Wallace presents, in layperson's language, both the history and the latest developments in this research. He lucidly pre-sents a world view based on Maharishi's Vedic Science which integrates the concepts of mind and body, consciousness and matter, and extends our concept of health beyond the individual to include the collective health of society.

Dr. Wallace's discussion brings out that in the Vedic understanding, the unified field of natural law—the most fundamental level of nature's intelligence—has always been described as a field of consciousness. This field underlies all physiological functioning, and can be accessed by the human mind. The direct experience of this field through tech-nologies of consciousness, including Transcendental Meditation, cre-ates balance throughout the physiology and is therefore essential in restoring a state of balance and health to the mind and body.

Maharishi Ayur-Ved—the ancient Vedic science of natural health care—emphasizes prevention of disease and promotion of health more than remedial medical intervention, through many cost-effective, natural approaches, including the technologies of consciousness. Eschewing modern medicine's narrow focus on disease, in which the wholeness of the patient's life in the context of society and the universe is lost, the approach outlined by Dr. Wallace heals the dualism of nineteenth-century science. The focus is instead on the promotion of optimal health and longevity as an essential element of higher states of consciousness, and on naturally avoiding diseases caused by unhealthy diet, lack of exercise, accumulation of stress, and other lifestyle factors.

From the perspective of a theoretical physicist with a deep interest in unified quantum field theories, Maharishi's Vedic Science is an unprecedented achievement. It is a complete science of consciousness and a comprehensive understanding of the laws of nature. Over the last five years, I have travelled to more than 35 countries to discuss science, technology and public policy with scientists and government leaders; campaigned as the presidential candidate of the Natural Law Party; and now am Director of the Institute of Science, Technology and Public Policy at Maharishi International University. Based on this experience, I believe that Maharishi's Vedic Science and Technology provides the most practical and realistic solution to the critical problems of individual and collective health.

I commend Dr. Wallace for what I believe to be both a fascinating story and an important source of vital knowledge. As consumers and providers of health care, we all stand to benefit from Dr. Wallace's work. *The Physiology of Consciousness* is essential reading for anyone who wants to develop perfect health and enjoy life in the highest state of human development.

DISCOVERING
OUR INNER PHYSIOLOGY

I T HAD TAKEN MORE THAN THREE YEARS OF RESEARCH TO PREPARE for the day I walked down the dimly lit underground corridor that led to the historic Thorndike Memorial Laboratory. The high standards of science practiced in this building were at odds with their surroundings. The Thorndike lab is situated in Boston City Hospital, a network of old, decaying buildings that might be mistaken for a foundling home out of a Dickens novel. Outside was what had become the worst of Boston ghettos. However, I was quickly given to understand that, as a medical researcher, I should take Puritan pride in the dingy setting; it was a badge of honor.

My heart pounded as I walked into the small lecture hall crowded with senior research scientists and medical doctors, the elite of Boston's medical community. I was not worried about the topic of my lecture, which was my Ph.D. thesis research. What was going to be difficult to communicate was the implications of that research. For the first time, a fourth state of consciousness, different from waking, dreaming, and sleeping—a state of pure consciousness—was readily accessible to science. This enormous breakthrough had been made possible by the introduction of an entirely new technology, a technology of consciousness. This technology, the Transcendental Meditation technique of

1

Maharishi Mahesh Yogi, systematically produced in those who practiced it the repeatable experience of pure consciousness. Studying the objective, physiological correlates of Transcendental Meditation, scientists could thus begin to pinpoint the physiology of consciousness.

I wanted this audience to understand that this was a turning point in the history of mankind. Two divergent streams of knowledge were converging. On the one hand, through the objective approach of modern science we were delving into the deepest layers of life and matter. In physiology, we had made enormous breakthroughs in our understanding of the relationship between mind and body. In physics we were on the verge of arriving at a single unified theory of matter and energy—Einstein's great dream. On the other hand, through a new subjective approach to gaining knowledge, we had for the first time a reliable and systematic means to explore the finest levels of our consciousness.

This subjective approach had been brought to light from the timeless Vedic tradition by Maharishi and was proving to be of immense importance to the scientific community. This approach and the new technology of consciousness it offered would entirely change our way of thinking about health and the human body.

The new area of research I was describing that day revealed that underlying our manifest, material physiology is a more fundamental, unmanifest physiology of consciousness. Understanding the physiology of consciousness gives us a new way of understanding and achieving ideal health, not only for the individual, but for the whole society.

The Biochemistry of Mind

My lecture at Thorndike Memorial Laboratory took place over twenty years ago, at a time when mind-body research was rapidly developing. Since then enormous changes have taken place, both in my own areas of research as well as in many others. Critical studies, especially in biochemistry, have helped uncover the connections between mind and body.

We can think of the body as having its own natural pharmacy. When we have a thought or feeling, the body responds by producing chemicals. These chemicals, which are produced in numerous types of cells, act as natural drugs that are involved in many different kinds of physiological and behavioral responses. One of the most interesting and widely publicized recent discoveries is that our mind can instruct our body to produce its own internal painkillers—a group of small protein compounds, or neuropeptides—called endorphins and enkephalins.

For many years researchers have been trying to find the cause of morphine and heroin addiction. In the course of their research, they isolated a particular receptor that seems specifically designed for morphine-type drugs. Receptors are biological molecules embedded on the surface of a cell. Specific hormones or chemicals in the blood and fluid surrounding the cell fit into specific receptors, the way a key fits into a lock. This sets off a chain of events inside the cell that results in a specific physiological action, such as an increase in metabolism.

The morphine molecule fits into certain receptors in the cells of the nervous system which, when activated, greatly reduce pain. Since morphine is a painkiller not normally present in the body, one could reasonably assume that nature designed these receptors for a substance that does exist in the body. That is to say, the body must have its own painkiller. Pursuing this logic, researchers were indeed able to identify painkillers produced by the body and to map their pathways throughout the brain and physiology. These painkillers, endorphins and enkephalins, also play a number of other important roles as "biological communicators." One of their most significant roles is to initiate the placebo effect.

A placebo induces the expectation of a pleasing effect, such as relief from pain, and this expectation itself causes the patient to actually experience less pain. It is well known that when subjects in an experiment are told they are being given a new painkilling drug and are instead given a white sugar pill with no active painkilling ingredient—a placebo—a large proportion of these people will not feel any pain, even when subjected to a moderately painful stimulus. For many years no one had any reasonable explanation for how the placebo worked—it was in fact considered a nuisance to scientific research, making it necessary to include more control subjects.

Experiments now suggest that the placebo effect is an important scientific breakthrough vividly illustrating the power of the mind over the body. The findings suggest that, in the placebo effect, the mind—convinced it will not feel pain—causes the nervous system to produce endorphins and enkephalins. The result is similar to taking a painkilling drug. One of the most interesting findings about endorphins and enkephalins is that their receptors have been located not only in the nervous system, where we generally think of pain and emotions as being processed, but in many other cells (for example, in the cells of the immune system).

We may consider the neuropeptide molecule and its cousin, the neurotransmitter, to be "precipitated thoughts." If we have an excited thought, then a molecule such as adrenaline arises and stimulates various parts of the body. If we have a calm, soothing thought, then a "calm" molecule arises—that is, one that produces a restful effect on the body. Such molecules form an information network through which any part of the body can "talk" to any other part. From this perspective, our body is a thinking body, in which information or intelligence constantly flows among all its innumerable parts.

This gives rise to the concept of an entirely subjective physiology of consciousness, which underlies our objective physiology of matter. The connection between the two is at the molecular level, where thoughts are translated into chemical messengers. Moment by moment the body is being influenced and changed—is actually being created—by the fluctuations of consciousness projected in our thoughts and feelings. Understood in this way, the mind-body connection has countless ramifications for biomedical research and practice, including the treatment of pain and serious disease.

The Discovery of the Unified Field
of All the Laws of Nature

The recent achievements in mind-body research have paralleled breakthroughs in modern physics. In physics, matter and energy are viewed as expressions of four fundamental fields: gravity, electromagnetism, and the strong and weak nuclear forces. In the last few years quantum physics has reached such a profound level of understanding that it has been able to locate one unified field of all the laws of nature at the basis of these four fields. While the complete mathematical description of this field is still developing, it is clear that the unified field of natural law is the source of all material diversity. It transcends all existence; it is a field of pure information from which all the different forces and laws of nature sequentially emerged in the first microseconds of the creation of our universe, and from which this process is continually taking place at every moment.

Most striking, modern physics' description of the unified field of natural law as a self-sufficient, self-interacting field of infinite intelligence and dynamism is remarkably similar to descriptions of the unified basis of creation given by the world's most ancient traditions of knowledge. In the Vedic tradition of India, all the diversity of material existence has always been described as sequentially emerging from a unified field, a self-sufficient, self-referral, unbounded and infinitely dynamic field of intelligence. As we will see, in the Vedic understanding this unified field of natural law is, in fact, defined as a field of pure intelligence, pure information in its most compact and concentrated form—one unified basis of life.

This concept of one unified field of natural law at the basis of creation is found in many cultural traditions of both East and West. With the advent of modern science some three hundred years ago, these ancient ideas lost their prominence and were eventually displaced by the classical view of physics—the classical paradigm.

According to Newtonian classical physics, the world is made of tiny, indestructible atoms. Matter is solid and easily measured. This viewpoint has permeated every academic discipline and every area of society, and has had an enormous impact on our world view.

With the development of quantum physics some 70 years ago, the classical paradigm has been gradually replaced by the quantum paradigm. In the world of quantum physics, matter is no longer solid; it is only a perturbation, a condensation in an underlying field. The famous Heisenberg uncertainty principle states that we can only know either the position or momentum of a particle, never both at the same time. In the quantum world, paradoxes abound. For example, particles may appear sometimes as particles and sometimes as waves. Even when we describe a particle, it is only in terms of "probability amplitudes," a mathematical description of a wave or field that states the statistical chance of defining either its location or momentum.

Quantum principles also challenge many commonly held beliefs and assumptions. For example, in the classical view, which is the realm of our daily experience, there is an objective world independent of the perceiver. This world is made up of clumps of matter separated from each other in time and space. Mind is separate from matter and is confined to the brain. As humans, we are self-contained independent entities; we are physical machines that have somehow learned to think.

From the quantum point of view, however, the objective world is composed of energy fields that arise from one unified quantum field. The reason behind the Heisenberg uncertainty principle is that the act of measuring affects the precision of measurement of the position or momentum of the particle. The objective world is thus no longer independent of the perceiver. And human beings are also not independent entities; we are focal points of intelligence in the unified field, inseparably interconnected with the patterns of intelligence which make up the entire universe. Our bodies are changing patterns of intelligence.

But do these principles ultimately have meaning for human life? One could argue that they make no sense because they have no relation to the "real world" of our everyday lives. Yet according to modern physics, the quantum world is more fundamental than the classical world. We can think of the foundation of a house, hidden from view beneath the ground. Without this foundation, the house cannot stand. The quantum world is the foundation of the classical world. Without the quantum world, the classical world would not exist.

Further, the radical new concepts of quantum physics, while defying our sensory experience and rational explanations of the world, give us access to new realms of applied technology. Quantum principles are an essential part of our computer and electronic age. They make possible the miracles of modern technology and reveal the hidden, underlying power and intelligence stored within matter. Matter has thus given way to information. It is easy to understand why it has taken so long for these ideas to be introduced to the general public—they challenged the belief in matter. They broke the boundaries of the classical paradigm and presented reality from an entirely different viewpoint.

The Vedic Paradigm

These advances in modern physics have coincided with Maharishi's reformulation of the knowledge and technology of consciousness from the Vedic tradition. What distinguishes the Vedic viewpoint from that of modern physics? Modern physics has grown to rely on the objective

6

method of gaining knowledge, which has touched upon, but has not uncovered the true nature of the observer himself—the very consciousness of the scientist. Despite the philosophical implications of quantum measurement theory (regarding the attention of the scientist), whole areas of vital knowledge concerning the subjective nature of consciousness have been neglected precisely because the objective approach could not reliably probe them.

Into the narrow intellectual atmosphere created by the dominance of modern science based approaches, Maharishi has boldly introduced a new paradigm, the Vedic paradigm. This world view restores the fundamental understanding that consciousness is the basic field of life. It is derived from Maharishi's revitalization of the profound wealth of Vedic wisdom. The manner in which he has brought this wisdom to light is of inestimable importance to mankind. He has taken a thoroughly modern and scientific angle to create a new science, his Vedic Science and Technology, which unifies the two polarities of the subjective and objective approaches to gaining knowledge. He has also encouraged scientists and scholars around the world to investigate, substantiate, and express Vedic wisdom using the terminology and technology of modern science.

As this book unfolds we will explore in detail Maharishi's explanation of the rich field of Vedic knowledge about the unified field of all the laws of nature, particularly as it relates to our understanding of physiology and health. Here I will simply summarize a few important principles; later on, each point will be considered more thoroughly.

When we say "natural law," we mean that intelligence which administers the whole universe, which right now is administering the functioning of our entire physiology, our heartbeat, our breathing, our brain wave activity, the activity of all the people on the earth, of the whole field of nature, and of the entire universe. This is natural law— it is an extraordinary intelligence, an infinite intelligence, which has infinite creativity and infinite organizing power. It is constantly and perpetually throughout time administering the evolution of the whole universe.

Both modern science and Maharishi's Vedic Science describe the fundamental state of all the natural laws operating throughout the entire universe as the unified field of natural law—the basic, self-interacting, unlimited field of nature's intelligence—the single, universal source of all the orderliness in nature. The unified field is the level of the total intelligence of nature.

Not only is this field the basis of all natural law; it creates from within itself all the diverse laws of nature governing life at every level of the manifest universe. How does it do this? The unified field of natural law is not static—again, it is a lively, self-interacting field of intelligence. It interacts within itself, and the dynamics of its self-interaction give rise to a process of precise sequential unfoldment of the laws of nature.

One major difference between Vedic Science and modern science is that in the Vedic paradigm, the foundation level of natural law is not only a field of pure intelligence. It is also a field of pure wakefulness or *pure consciousness*—consciousness fully awake within itself—which Maharishi also describes as a state of pure singularity.

Thus Maharishi's Vedic Science describes the self-interacting dynamics of the unified field as the eternal dynamics of consciousness knowing itself. From this self-interaction within the unified field of pure consciousness, the laws of nature begin to unfold. As they unfold, they take form as the expressions of *pure knowledge*, known in Maharishi's Vedic Science as the *Ved*. The same fundamental laws of nature described mathematically in the unified quantum field theories of modern physics are embodied in the structure of the Rik Ved, the most fundamental aspect of the Vedic literature.

In the Vedic paradigm, the unified field is therefore not only the source of matter, but also—because it is pure consciousness—the source of mind. It is the common source of mind and body, of subjective experience and material creation. Consciousness is therefore the underlying field from which matter arises. Further, the investigation of the unified field of natural law is not confined to intellectual analysis; this field can be directly experienced through the subjective technologies of consciousness Maharishi has brought to light from the Vedic literature.

Maharishi has recently referred to the Rik Ved as the Constitution of the Universe. We don't usually think of the universe as having a constitution. But every body of laws, whether manmade or nature's laws, must originate from some underlying, unifying principles. Just as the constitution of a nation represents the most fundamental level of national law and the basis of all the laws governing the nation, the Rik Ved, the Constitution of the Universe, represents the most fundamental level of natural law and the basis of all known laws of nature.

Maharishi defines the Constitution of the Universe as "the eternal, non-changing basis of natural law and the ultimate source of the order and harmony displayed throughout creation." This level of nature, he says, is lively in the intelligence of every grain of creation.

In a later chapter, we will look more fully into Maharishi's discovery of the Constitution of the Universe. We will examine the dynamics of how the laws of nature unfold from within the unified field, and appreciate the precise mathematical correspondence between the two descriptions of this process in modern science and Maharishi's Vedic Science. Most important, we will see not only why it is valuable to understand the Constitution of the Universe, but why it is crucial for us to actually experience and enliven this level of nature's intelligence in our own minds, so that its total potential can be lived in human life.

The further implications of the Vedic paradigm are even more significant. Not only does it bring new, unforeseen depth to the study of human physiology. It gives us the ability to reconnect individual life with its foundation in the unified field of natural law, so that life can be lived in accord with all the laws of nature.

A Technology of Consciousness

When I stood before my audience at Thorndike laboratory some twenty years ago, I knew it would be nearly impossible to communicate the importance and impact of this new paradigm. As the quantum paradigm led to the introduction of radically new and more powerful technologies at the electronic and nuclear layers of matter, the Vedic paradigm introduces even more powerful technologies in the realm of consciousness.

In the lecture I presented my first studies on the Transcendental Meditation technique, one of the primary subjective technologies of the Vedic paradigm introduced by Maharishi. I had been studying the objective correlates of Transcendental Meditation, attempting to physiologically define the fourth major state of consciousness—transcendental or pure consciousness. While there are many techniques of meditation and self-development, my research and personal experience had shown conclusively that Transcendental Meditation was the most systematic and reliable for producing consistent physiological correlates of pure consciousness.

In presenting the results of my research to this audience, I realized that to them, the existence of transcendental consciousness could only be appreciated and understood in terms of its objective physiological correlates—heart rate, blood lactate, skin resistance. Yet I knew that, exciting as these findings were, they were only the shadowy reflections of the incomparable richness of the transcendental field of life—the deep mechanics of natural law unfolding within pure consciousness, reverberating unsuspected within these very doctors' own consciousness.

If the real nature of life is a unified field of consciousness, why don't we experience it as the reality of our daily lives? Why do we experience the world as being made of separate material objects: why does our body, for example, appear to be localized in time and space? The reasons is that our senses are highly selective. The senses are activated by a narrow spectrum of data from the immense flux of nature, and it is from a selection of that narrow spectrum that our understanding of physical reality is determined.

Our nervous system constructs our reality. The nervous system analyzes the world in terms of patterns of sight, sound, taste, touch, and smell, and then our mind and intellect actively reconstruct within the brain our individual perception of reality. The reason we experience the world from a classical perspective, in which matter appears solid, is that we do not have access to the deeper levels of reality beyond the obvious sensory level of experience.

We have not learned to use the full potential of our nervous system to directly experience and explore the wide range of nature's intelligence; we have been forced to rely on the vision provided for us by objective technology alone. This limited awareness, using only objective means, has led us to know only the grosser aspects of our physiology of matter, which embody a tiny fraction of the laws of nature.

To gain a true picture of the world, we must first use the full abilities of the nervous system to experience consciousness in its simplest state, the state of pure consciousness, the unified field of natural law.

Through the subjective technologies of Maharishi's Vedic Science, the focus of attention is periodically shifted inward. We begin to use our nervous sytem as a special kind of microscope with which to explore pure consciousness in a systematic and reliable way. This experience cultures our nervous system to function in a more integrated and coherent style.

As a natural and spontaneous result of this experience, our preconditioned interpretation of the world—and the belief system we have built from it—begins to change. With the regular, direct experience of the unified field, our conscious experience and intellect are no longer restricted by the belief that matter is the only reality. We experience a new reality, of pure consciousness at the basis of matter.

We know this not intellectually, but through direct experience. We know it first as the field of pure consciousness at the basis of our own mind. As our practice of these technologies advances, we develop towards higher states of consciousness, and come to know pure consciousness as the field underlying everything we encounter through our senses in the world around us. Our nervous system then constructs for us a reality far richer, more delightful and fulfilling than the one we were accustomed to when the classical viewpoint dominated our sensory experience. Eventually we gain access within our own consciousness to the source of nature's creativity, the Ved, the dynamic processes that structure the universe. We are no longer separate from nature. As consciousness becomes fully developed, we can look forward to experiencing our inner Self as the consciousness of the universe.

The unified field is one single, universal field underlying—transcendental to—all existence. Yet within this transcendental field of unity exists the Rik Ved, the Constitution of the Universe, like a beautiful fabric containing innumerable permutations or patterns. Modern science calls these patterns "the laws of nature." In the Vedic paradigm, however, these laws or patterns are not seen as isolated material phenomena; on the contrary, they are woven into the fabric of pure consciousness itself.

The implications of the Vedic paradigm are far-reaching. They are found in every area of life. This knowledge is applied in the field of health and medicine, for example, through the complete system of health care known as Maharishi Ayur-Ved, which will be discussed at length in this book. The theoretical basis of Maharishi Ayur-Ved is found in Maharishi's Vedic Physiology, which includes a complete understanding of the relationship between mind and body.

The fundamental premise of Maharishi's Vedic Physiology is that mind and body are both expressions of the laws of nature within one unified field, the unified field of pure consciousness. All aspects of physiology are studied in light of their emergence from, and connection to, the unified field of pure consciousness.

Vedic Physiology includes four primary divisions. The study of our *physiology of consciousness* includes the mind and all mental phenomena. The *physiology of matter* includes study of the fundamental structures of natural law as they emerge from pure consciousness, and the hierarchical structure of the nervous system and the body. The *physiology of society* extends beyond our individual body to include the collective consciousness of society. Finally, the *physiology of the universe* encompasses everything from the Ved—the fine fabrics of natural law, the impulses of intelligence at the basis of creation—to its expressions in the entire universe. These divisions are somewhat arbitrary, since everything in the universe is an expression of the unified field of natural law, the field of pure consciousness. However, I have found these categories to be useful for purposes of discussion.

The concepts of Vedic Physiology have not only profound theoretical significance, but immense practical benefits for the unfoldment of our full mental and physical potential and for improving the quality of life in society. As a physiologist for over twenty years, I see the emergence of Maharishi's Vedic Physiology as a fundamental discovery in our understanding of the potential of the human body and brain. For the first time, on the basis of this knowledge, we will be able to fully realize the power of human consciousness. We can reconnect individual life with the life of the cosmos, with the evolutionary power of nature, and become the lively embodiment of natural law.

These were the ideas I attempted to express in my lecture so many years ago. If we are able to experience the full range of consciousness, the restrictions on our awareness are removed: we transcend the myth of matter and gain a complete and unified understanding of life. As Louis Pasteur, one of the great founders of modern medicine and physiology, wrote:

You place matter before life and you decide that matter has existed for all eternity. How do you know that the incessant progress of Science will not compel scientists to consider that life has existed during eternity, and not matter? You pass from matter to life because your intelligence of today cannot conceive things otherwise. How do you know that in ten thousand years one will not consider it more likely that matter has emerged from life?

PART 1

THE PHYSIOLOGY
OF CONSCIOUSNESS

CHAPTER 1

THE ANATOMY
OF CONSCIOUSNESS

I N 1974 I FLEW WITH A PHYSICIST FRIEND TO NEPAL. WE MADE
our way up from Katmandu, the capital, to be nearer the
Himalayas, and found a beautiful alpine lake, which Nepalese
princes once favored as a summer retreat. For less than a dollar,
we rented a small boat and pushed out onto the water. It was a windy
day with clearing skies, a perfect day to fly kites. I had bought one at
the bazaar. It was painted a fierce red and built for acrobatics. As I
stood up in the boat and let the kite loose on the wind, it jumped from
my hand. Children ran along the shore, laughing and waving to us.

The kite floated high into the thin air. I remember looking up
toward the great mountains around us. Though they were mostly covered with clouds, they gave off an aura of grandeur and peace. I felt content, almost drowsy, in this moment of ease. As I watched, the clouds
lifted all at once. I was absolutely in awe. What I had taken for mountains were only foothills! Beyond, like ancient gods, rose the true
Himalayas, unbelievably mighty and majestic.

So much power and beauty were concentrated in that breathtaking
scene that my friend and I could hardly speak. The name of one of the
tallest peaks is Annapurna, which means "fullness of life." And what I
experienced in that moment was a feeling of utter fulfillment and

17

unboundedness, a simple yet profound conviction that time really is timeless, and that anything is possible.

The Himalayas are the home of the Vedic tradition of India, and people have always journeyed there seeking enlightenment and immortality. In the Vedic tradition, enlightenment represents the ultimate development of what we consider the most valuable qualities of human life. It is something real and natural. It develops continuously, progressively, and systematically on the basis of neurophysiological refinement utilizing the full potential of human physiology.

Throughout the world I have found a genuine interest, among serious scientists and laypeople alike, in consciousness and enlightenment. Everywhere, there is the growing recognition that we have neglected the subjective development of life and have become too obsessed with material development. We understand in great detail the anatomy of matter; it is now time to focus on the anatomy of consciousness.

Understanding the Nature of Consciousness

The modern approach to understanding the nature of consciousness has been largely the domain of psychology. As objective matter is the principal topic of physics, subjective consciousness is the principal topic of psychology—or at least it should be. Early in the history of experimental psychology, scientists recognized that subjective reports of conscious experiences were highly variable. It was difficult, if not impossible, to use the objective methodology of science to study what was apparently highly subjective.

From this vacuum of reliable experimental data arose the field of behaviorism. Behaviorism avoided studying the subjective mind; instead, it focused entirely on measurable behavior. Behaviorism dominated psychology for many years primarily because it allowed psychologists to become a part of the existing paradigm of materialism. Materialism is the name given to the contemporary scientific viewpoint that regards living organisms as purely physio-chemical machines; it stems from the understanding that consciousness is an epiphenomenon—that is, it arises as the by-product of the functioning of a complex nervous system.

The emphasis in psychology for many years now has been in cognitive psychology, which is concerned mainly with information processing and selective attention. Dr. David Orme-Johnson, director of the doctoral program in psychology at Maharishi International University (MIU) in Fairfield, Iowa, comments on this phenomenon. (MIU is the leading center in North America for teaching and research developing the connections between Maharishi's Vedic Science and Technology and modern academic fields of knowledge). Dr. Orme-Johnson points out that while cognitive psychology is an improvement over behaviorism, like so many other trends in psychology it has given us no real insight into the nature of consciousness.

He notes that psychologists collectively generate over 100 research articles per day and have published about 800,000 articles since the first volume of *Psychological Abstracts* appeared in 1927. Studies have shown, however, that very little practical knowledge has come from this volume of research. As the authors of one study concluded: "The failure of the social sciences to produce many pragmatically important products would be perhaps tragic were it not for the fact that the world has survived and will likely continue to survive without them."

From the perspective of the Vedic paradigm, Dr. Orme-Johnson explains, modern psychology's major shortcoming is its lack of a systematic technology to directly experience the state of pure consciousness, the basis of the mind and the foundation for all mental processes. Owing to this lack, psychology has focused primarily on the "classical" or active, content-oriented level of the mind; it has not addressed the underlying unity of the "quantum" or unmanifest, unbounded level of the mind. As a result, there is still no complete unified theory in psychology.

The Three-in-One Structure of Consciousness

What we consider to be ordinary waking consciousness is a very restricted value of the full range of human consciousness. It corresponds with the more active levels of human life. Systematically quieting the internal functioning of the physiology while enlivening the deeper levels of mental awareness allows us to experience the fourth state of consciousness—a much fuller and more universal state of consciousness—one that is completely awake, yet settled and unified.

This is a description of what happens during Maharishi's Transcendental Meditation technique, and in the Vedic paradigm, this unified state of consciousness is referred to as *transcendental consciousness*. It is the experience of pure consciousness, the unified field of natural law, the transcendental field of life. To experience this state, our attention has been brought from the active, surface level of thinking to the silent, unbounded ocean of consciousness at the basis of the mind. In the experience of pure consciousness, there are no thoughts, no sensory experience, and no distinction between subject and object—only pure awareness, the experience of consciousness knowing itself.

As I said earlier, in Maharishi's Vedic Science this field of pure consciousness is also described as a field of pure wakefulness—consciousness fully awake within itself. It is a field of pure intelligence, and being intelligent, it knows itself. When pure consciousness, by virtue of being "conscious," knows or becomes aware of itself—becomes awake within its own nature—it remains in its unified state, yet appears as three different modes of consciousness: pure consciousness (the *knower*) knows itself as pure consciousness (the *known*) through the instrumentality of pure consciousness (the *process of knowing*). Thus pure consciousness is described as having a unified, "three-in-one" structure. As Maharishi explains:

"This structure is very easy to understand. The awareness is open to itself, and therefore the awareness knows itself. Because the awareness knows itself it is the knower, it is the known, and it is the process of knowing. This is the state of pure intelligence, wide-awake in its own nature and completely self-referral. This is pure consciousness, transcendental consciousness."

Because pure consciousness is the basis of all the other levels of the mind, its basic three-in-one structure is found at every level of human experience. To help us understand the concept better, let's momentarily step out of the abstract field of pure consciousness, and see how the knower, process of knowing, and known are the components of experiences we are all familiar with in ordinary waking consciousness.

When you see any object—a rose, for instance—there are three modes of your experience. There is you, the knower; the rose, the known; and the connection between you and the rose, the processes of perception or knowing. This structure works differently in waking consciousness, however, from the way it does in the state of pure consciousness. When you experience the rose in waking consciousness,

20

your awareness becomes identified with it, and the knower becomes overshadowed. Only the rose, the object of knowing, is lively in your experience.

In waking consciousness we can talk about a flower as an object of our experience. Going back to the state of pure consciousness, however, what do we find? Our processes of perception have turned within to experience our own inner nature. We can't talk in terms of the rose as an object of experience, because it is an object only in the outer world. When we are experiencing pure consciousness, the rose simply does not exist for us. There is only the unified value of consciousness, in which pure consciousness, the knower, is the sole object of its own knowing. For this reason pure consciousness is also described as *self-referral* consciousness. It is the unified experience of knower, process of knowing, and known, in which consciousness is awake to its full unbounded nature as the Self, the unmanifest source of all creation

Consciousness knowing itself: this three-in-one structure is the beginning point of the self-interacting dynamics of pure consciousness. From this simple coexistence of one and three—of unity and diversity—the process of unfoldment of natural law, the Ved, begins. The self-interacting dynamics continues to unfold, and through all the transformations that arise during this process are created the laws of nature that govern the entire universe.

The goal of Maharishi's Vedic Physiology is to enliven this unified state of consciousness, the unified field of all the laws of nature, in our own awareness using specific mental technologies, so that the fundamental laws governing human physiology and all of life everywhere become fully lively in our life. Physicists can make a simple change at the quantum level of the atom to unleash tremendous power at the classical level of the objective world. Likewise, by enlivening pure consciousness, the level of the Constitution of the Universe, we can make simple changes at the fundamental quantum level of our physiology of consciousness, and thus create dramatic changes at the classical level of our physiology of matter.

This possibility has tremendous implications for the fields of psychology, physiology, and the health sciences; as we shall see later on, it is the basis for creating ideal health for the individual and ideal health for the whole society—a state of irreversible world peace. To better understand its mechanics, let's first examine the basic anatomy of our consciousness.

The Structures of the Physiology of Consciousness

The basic anatomy of consciousness consists of five mental structures. The most fundamental level is the unbounded field of pure consciousness. This is the state of pure singularity or pure wakefulness, the unified three-in-one state of knower, process of knowing, and known. This is our Self, the foundation level of individual consciousness and individual life.

At the risk of being overly repetitive, I want to emphasize that this field of pure consciousness at the deepest level of the human mind is the same universal field of pure consciousness at the basis of all existence. It is the unified field of all the laws of nature. The Self of our own existence is also the most fundamental level of subjectivity in nature. Thus the structures of the physiology of consciousness—in fact, all the dynamics and elements we describe here in relation to pure consciousness—are not only found at the basis of individual life, but are the broad principles and structures of natural law at the foundation of everything in creation.

Here I want to introduce a few new terms from Sanskrit, the language of Maharishi's Vedic Science—in Maharishi's words, "the language of nature"—that precisely describe the mechanics and dynamics of this field. In the three-in-one structure of pure consciousness knowing itself, the knower is called *Rishi*, the process of knowing is *Devata*, and the known is *Chhandas*. The unified state, the togetherness value or "collectedness" of knower, process of knowing, and known, is called *Samhita*.

It may help us understand these new terms to see that they also relate to our experience of concrete objects in the waking state. Because they are universal principles found at every level of creation, we can find Rishi, Devata, and Chhandas at even this most concrete level.

Going back again to pure consciousness, we find once more that the dynamics of Rishi, Devata, and Chhandas are different from their nature in the waking state. At this level, Rishi, Devata, and Chhandas are not three separate aspects of experience. There is no distinction between subject and object: again, the knower is the sole object of its own knowing. Thus the three are found in one unified, self-interacting state. It is this unified experience of knower, process of knowing, and known that Maharishi refers to as "the Samhita of Rishi, Devata, and Chhandas."

Maharishi explains that the Samhita, or unity value of pure consciousness, is eternal and unbroken. Why, then, do diversified values appear within it? Because the intelligence value of pure consciousness, in observing its own unity, "conceptually locates" within itself the three values of knower, process of knowing, and known—Rishi, Devata, and Chhandas.

But each of the three is essentially just a mode of the one pure consciousness. To state this a different way, each of these three values is, in Maharishi's terms, an "intellectual construct" arising from the self-referral activity of consciousness observing itself, within the eternal, unbroken continuum of pure consciousness.

Maharishi often refers to pure consciousness as the "sea of consciousness," or the "unbounded ocean of consciousness" at the unmanifest basis of creation. He refers to the coexistence of the three and the one unified state as "the first principle of nature's functioning," the primary and most fundamental expression of nature's dynamics. And in the internal dynamics of this field—in this elementary relationship of Rishi, Devata, and Chhandas in pure consciousness—is seated the primordial power of nature, the total potential of natural law.

The self-interacting dynamics does not stop, however, with the emergence of this three-in-one structure. The process continues. From the primary interaction of Samhita of Rishi, Devata, and Chhandas—pure consciousness knowing itself—come many other relationships and interactions.

Now we are entering into a very refined area in the realm of Maharishi's Vedic Science. In Chapters 13 and 14, as I promised earlier, we are going to look more thoroughly into the extraordinary details of what happens as natural law begins to unfold within pure consciousness. For now, we will merely sketch the process according to Maharishi's explanation in fairly general terms.

In the process of conceptualizing itself as the different values of Rishi, Devata, and Chhandas, pure consciousness becomes transformed.

Different permutations and combinations of Samhita, Rishi, Devata, and Chhandas begin to be created, and this produces further transformations or fluctuations within pure consciousness. The self-interacting dynamics of consciousness continues, endlessly multiplying itself and creating countless transformations. Actually, what is created is a *series* of transformations that unfolds in a set, precise, and perfectly orderly sequence.

Maharishi comments that "innumerable values of the knower, the known, and the process of knowing are contained in that sea of consciousness," constituting the "innumerable qualities of self-interaction in the self-referral state of consciousness." All these different specific values of Rishi, Devata, and Chhandas, and all the processes of transformation among them, form an eternal continuum at the unmanifest basis of creation.

From this continuum of self-interacting dynamics of the sea of consciousness, the laws of nature spontaneously emerge that give rise to the entire universe. The sequential transformations of the mutual relationships among Rishi, Devata, and Chhandas are expressed as the fundamental laws of nature. And this, in the Vedic paradigm, is how the whole creation sequentially unfolds in a precise and beautiful manner.

The ocean of consciousness is a field of infinite silence. And yet, as we might expect from the phenomenal level of transformations constantly taking place within it, it is also a field of tremendous potential dynamism. This is how Maharishi describes it: "The self-referral state of pure consciousness is an infinitely dynamic, inexhaustible source of energy and creativity. On that basis the whole creation goes on perpetually in its infinite variety, multiplying itself all the time."

As the transformations progress, the intelligence aspect of pure consciousness continues to discriminate, until all possible transformations of its own nature are exhausted. Eventually the laws of nature take concrete form: matter emerges, the concrete structures of the physiology of creation, and from that the infinite diversity of the whole universe.

In Maharishi's explanation, the Vedic literature is the "script" of this process of sequential unfoldment of the perfectly orderly structure of natural law that governs the whole process of creation and evolution in nature. It displays the total knowledge of the primordial power of nature structured in the internal dynamics of the sea of consciousness.

Now that we've had an overview of the finest mechanics of nature emerging from within pure consciousness, it's legitimate for us to ask how this relates to human life. How do we fit into this picture?

The Levels of the Mind

The infinite dynamism of pure consciousness is the source of all structures of natural law in the entire universe, which means in our life as well. All that we just described is eternally going on at the basis of creation, within the field of pure consciousness—*our own* field of pure consciousness. This self-referral field, the total potential of nature's intelligence, is at the basis of our own life. Having understood this, we can now consider how the levels of subjectivity unfold in individual life from pure consciousness, the Self.

The self-interacting dynamics of consciousness ultimately structure all mental and material phenomena. Sequentially unfolding from pure consciousness, what first arise are the mental phenomena (the more expressed levels of the physiology of consciousness), and then the hierarchical structure of the physiology of matter.

The basic level of the mind is the Self, the universal field of pure consciousness. From the Self, the next levels of subjectivity arise—ego, intellect, mind, and senses. The ego is the deepest level of individuality. Here resides the faintest level of feeling, which involves intuition and the individual's basic values. The third level is the intellect, which is responsible for discrimination. The intellect functions both as a decision-maker and as a controller for selective attention. Arising from the intellect is the fourth level, the mind. (In Maharishi's Vedic Science, the term "mind" in its broadest sense refers to all the levels of the subjective physiology. Here, however, "mind" refers to that mental structure which is concerned with memory and association.) At the fifth and most expressed level are the five senses, which process all incoming information from their environment.

These structures are common to all human beings. The level of the Self is a universal structure that underlies the other four levels. The Self is the same, unbounded field of unlimited potential in everyone. However, the four expressed levels differ in content, or expression, from individual to individual. They arise from pure consciousness in the same way that the elementary particles are formed from energy and matter. In quantum physics, elementary particles are defined in terms of stable fluctuations of the underlying unified field. The subjective mental structures of consciousness may also be regarded as the major modes of expression arising from the patterns in the underlying field of pure consciousness.

The Vedic paradigm thus provides a complete understanding of the fundamental relationship between the subjective and objective spheres of creation: underlying all levels of consciousness and all expressions of matter is one unified field of natural law—one field of pure consciousness. Subjectivity and objectivity are not separate, discrete aspects of life, never to be reconciled; they are merely different themes of the same fundamental field of life.

Without this understanding, we are left with a fragmented view of ourselves and of nature. Without this understanding, practical applications for improving individual and social life must remain limited. By separating subjectivity from objectivity, we have disconnected ourselves from ourselves; we have lost the connection between the physiology of consciousness and the physiology of matter. The technologies of the Vedic paradigm are primarily subjective technologies that provide a systematic, reliable means to directly experience pure consciousness, the underlying basis of these layers of the mind, and thus to re-enliven this connection.

The single most important discovery within the Vedic paradigm is the identification of the unified field of natural law as the field of pure consciousness—the Self. In one stroke, this realization again unifies human life with nature. By understanding and experiencing pure consciousness, the finest level of the anatomy of consciousness, we not only enrich all the more expressed layers of our physiology of consciousness, but we also uncover and make lively in ourselves the deepest level of the mechanics of nature's creativity. We experience our own self-interacting dynamics of consciousness, which creates everything from within itself.

This most profound level of nature, within which reside all the fundamental forces that ultimately structure the entire universe, is also the most intimate level of our subjective existence—our own Being.

Higher States of Consciousness

The regular experience of pure consciousness refines our physiology of matter so that we are able to realize the full range of human development in higher states of consciousness.

Our understanding and experience of consciousness itself has been limited, because we have had access to only three states of consciousness: waking, dreaming, and sleeping. The Vedic paradigm delineates distinct higher states of consciousness and describes precisely how they develop through regular practice of the technologies of Maharishi's Vedic Science. If we don't have the tools to develop and experience higher states of consciousness, then we confine ourselves to an extremely limited experience and understanding of nature; we isolate ourselves from the very heart of our own existence.

Maharishi's Vedic Science gives us the understanding and experience of seven states of consciousness—the three we are all familiar with, plus pure consciousness and three distinct higher states. The first step toward higher states of consciousness is to experience the fourth state—pure consciousness. With the regular experience of pure consciousness during Transcendental Meditation, the nervous system adapts to a new style of functioning. The alternation of transcendental consciousness with the regular daily cycle of waking activity, dreaming, and sleep produces a gradual refinement of neurophysiological functions. This results in a fifth state of consciousness—a new, more expanded state known as *cosmic consciousness*.

In cosmic consciousness the individual realizes his essential identity as transcendental or pure consciousness as an all-time reality. In this fifth state, transcendental consciousness *coexists* with waking, dreaming, and sleep. For example, in cosmic consciousness, even in the most dynamic waking-state activity, one has an inner quality of consciousness that is restful and absolutely clear; even while sleeping, one experiences the inner alertness of transcendental consciousness. Maharishi refers to this all-time silent inner alertness, which is the experience of transcendental consciousness along with all the changing states of awareness, as "witnessing."

In cosmic consciousness, because the awareness is permanently established in the field of pure consciousness, the impressions made by an object upon the nervous system no longer overshadow the

27

knower. An analogy may help explain this. In ordinary waking consciousness, our experience of anything in the outside world—even a beautiful rose—is like etching a line in rock: it leaves a deep, long-lasting impression that is difficult to erase and overshadows the underlying nature of pure consciousness. Maharishi explains that in this phenomenon,

> the image of the flower travels to the retina of the eye and reaches the mind. The image of the flower impressed on the mind gives the experience of the flower. The result is that the mind, as it receives the impression of the flower, is overshadowed by that impression. The mind's essential nature is obscured; the image of the flower remains impressed on it. The observer, or the mind, is as though lost in the experience.

With the regular experience of transcending, however, pure consciousness rises more and more into the nature of the mind, and ordinary waking consciousness becomes transformed. And when cosmic consciousness is fully established, Maharishi explains,

> the impression will be there, because the flower will be seen, but it will be like a line on water. It is drawn, it is seen, and yet simultaneously erased. This is how the fullness of the state of Being [pure consciousness] is maintained, and at the same time the outside, objective experience is maintained.

Maharishi emphasizes that it is not by *thinking about* pure consciousness or by trying to maintain a mood or intellectual idea of pure consciousness in the mind while experiencing objects that the mind achieves this level of development. It is only by the simple process of transcending and *directly experiencing* pure consciousness that its nature spontaneously rises in the mind, giving us the experience of pure, unbounded bliss at the same time we are enjoying the exterior world to the maximum. Maharishi also makes the point that cosmic consciousness is not a state of withdrawal from life. Far from it, because the experience of pure consciousness increases the conscious capacity of the mind, and therefore our experience of objects becomes deeper, richer, and more substantial.

Maharishi describes how the continuing refinement of the neurophysiology results in two more advanced states of consciousness. In the sixth state, called *refined* or *glorified cosmic consciousness*, perception becomes so refined as to appreciate the finest values of every object of perception along with unbounded pure consciousness.

Whereas in cosmic consciousness the knower realizes his *essential nature* as pure consciousness, the sixth state involves the refinement of the more expressed values of the knower—the mechanisms of perception. One begins to perceive the subtler values of the object of perception. It is as if the qualities of pure consciousness, firmly established at the deepest level of subjectivity, begin to spill out into the objective world of what we see and hear.

The seventh state of consciousness, traditionally referred to as Unity consciousness, is the pinnacle of human development—complete enlightenment. In the state of unity, inner and outer realities are seen in terms of their most universal and unbounded nature—the Self. One knows pure consciousness to be the underlying reality not only of one's own subjective nature, but of every object of perception in the objective world. One comprehends change and nonchange, the two fundamental aspects of life, simultaneously and sees that they are nothing other than the expression of unbounded pure consciousness—the wholeness of the unified field of natural law moving within itself. Maharishi comments, "The enlightened man, while beholding and acting in the whole of diversified creation, does not fall from his steadfast Unity of life, with which his mind is saturated and which remains indelibly fused in his vision."

Maharishi emphasizes that the growth towards higher states of consciousness occurs naturally through the practice of Transcendental Meditation. Higher states are not experienced as something strange or bizarre; rather, we experience them as completely natural states of awareness.

From my own research, I am convinced that as scientists we need to explore more deeply the anatomy of consciousness and the patterns of development of higher states of consciousness. We have set our sights too low. By seeking knowledge of human life and health with a focus on the physiology of matter alone, we have raised our eyes only as far as the foothills. As the mountaineer Maurice Herzog said as he neared the peak of Annapurna,

> There was something unusual in the way I saw my companion and everything around us. . . . all sense of exertion was gone, as though

there were no longer any gravity. This diaphanous landscape, this quintessence of purity—these were not the mountains I knew: they were the mountains of my dreams.

When the clouds clear—that will be when we avail ourselves of all the knowledge that the Vedic paradigm has to offer, of both the finest mechanics of natural law in the Ved, and their immense practical applications for human life. This is nothing less than the complete understanding of health and human physiology—and when we know this, then we will know the high peaks in all their splendor.

CHAPTER 2

QUANTIFYING THE PATTERNS
OF TRANSCENDING

L EARNING TO TRANSCEND IS THE FIRST PREREQUISITE FOR studying the anatomy of consciousness. To transcend means to go beyond. In the case of Transcendental Meditation it means that the conscious mind goes beyond the limitations it experiences in the ordinary states of waking, dreaming, and sleep. Transcendental Meditation and the more advanced TM-Sidhi program are the principal technologies of the Vedic paradigm. In Transcendental Meditation, one transcends the ordinary excited levels of thinking—the boundaries of the mind—and experiences deeper, quieter, and more powerful levels of the thinking process. Eventually, even thinking is left behind, and the mind experiences the self-referral dynamics of the unbounded field of pure, transcendental consciousness.

Transcending is essential to Transcendental Meditation. One can read many elaborate, often obscure descriptions of various forms of meditation. However, Maharishi makes it clear that the single, inflexible criterion for any true form of meditation is that it enables the mind to settle into a state of deep silence while remaining awake—that is, to experience its basis in transcendental consciousness. Maharishi's restoration of the fundamental principle of transcending is fortunate for all human beings, and also for science.

We might ask, "If transcendental consciousness is such a desirable state, why has it been virtually ignored and disregarded by advanced Western society?" The principal reason is that a reliable, verifiable technology for experiencing transcendental consciousness has not been available. Without an effective technology to systematically refine mental activity, transcendental consciousness became merely an esoteric topic of discussion.

Imagine what would happen if the world somehow returned to a primitive state, but with all the machinery of modern technology left intact. After a few generations, without scientists or technicians to explain how a modern power station worked, the equipment would break down and become useless. Untrained in its use, people would eventually ignore it, and the knowledge it represented would become misinterpreted or simply disappear. Even a manual on how to repair the equipment would seem useless, or possibly even mystical, if one couldn't understand its technical jargon.

This analogy is not so different from what has transpired over millennia in many countries. Once there did exist very lively and effective traditions of gaining higher states of consciousness. Yet in India, as well as in other countries, they remained vital only as long as the people conscientiously followed the correct meditation procedures. Some traditions of knowledge were disrupted because of upheavals in the social or political structure. Historically, invasion and subsequent domination by an outside culture weakened the inner integrity of native culture and traditions. In some countries, particularly India and China, meditation was taught only to a select few monks; the common people, becoming too involved in the daily routine of living, neglected its practice. There may have been thousands of reasons for the decline of knowledge, but the overall result was that fewer and fewer people within the parent traditions continued to achieve and maintain higher states of consciousness.

Because only an isolated few were experiencing higher states, there was no common ground on which such experiences could be understood. The vast majority of people who were not living in higher states began doubting the entire method. Since it was inaccessible to them and to most other people, why should they believe the experience of a few older seers who lived apart from the mainstream of society? What was once regarded as the highest level of knowledge, the acme of truth and practical achievement, came to be regarded as mystical and impractical.

With Maharishi's revival of the correct methodology, it is now possible to systematically and repeatedly experience transcendental consciousness. Besides providing enormous practical benefits for the individual, this methodology has made it possible for us to experientially and experimentally explore the relationship between the physiology of consciousness and the physiology of matter in the development toward higher states of consciousness.

Research on Consciousness

In the Vedic paradigm, while consciousness is the basis of matter, consciousness requires the material physiology to support its activity. In order for the physiology of consciousness to act and develop, it needs the physiology of matter. Therefore, whenever the mind experiences transcendental consciousness—a subjective state of completely expanded awareness—something measurable must show up in the body at the same time.

Physiological recordings cannot tell us what the experience of transcendence feels like. But the patterns they display are a way of tracing the fingerprint that the state of transcendental consciousness leaves upon the body, both during and after the experience. By studying a wide range of physiological and biochemical parameters, we are perceiving the patterns in this fingerprint in increasingly fine detail. These patterns are one means we have of understanding and quantifying the fundamental patterns of nature's intelligence lively at the basis of human experience, and seeing how they affect the whole physiology and individual health.

Maharishi's introduction of the Transcendental Meditation technique to the West in the late 1950s made systematic research on consciousness possible for the first time. Because the technique is taught in a systematic and reliable way, the researcher is assured that all subjects are using the same procedure. And because instruction is available practically everywhere in the world, subjects are readily available.

From their first day of TM practice, individuals frequently report the effortless experience of a state of inner silence, inner wakefulness, and inner peace. The degree of clarity of the experience of transcendental consciousness may vary considerably, but everyone has a taste of it because of the inherent naturalness and effectiveness of the technique. Such experiences became the focal point for my initial research.

I began research in 1967 as a graduate student at the UCLA Physiology Department and Brain Research Institute. At the time I conducted the research, I had no idea of the impact it would have. Since then, there have been more than 500 studies conducted at 200 universities and independent research institutions in 30 countries on the effects of Transcendental Meditation and the TM-Sidhi program. This body of research includes publications in over 100 refereed journals.

The Physiological Patterns of
Transcendental Consciousness

A major finding that physiological studies on the TM technique have revealed is the unique state of "restful alertness" that subjects experience: the body settles down to a state of deep rest and relaxation, while the mind is fully awake and alert. During meditation, for example, subjects show a decrease in heart rate, respiration rate, oxygen consumption, and plasma cortisol and lactate levels, and an increase in skin resistance, phenylalanine levels, and EEG (electroencephalographic) coherence.

Many early studies took a general approach, comparing the average magnitude of a particular variable (such as respiration rate) during experimental and control periods. There was no attempt to isolate and characterize specific periods in which subjects were experiencing transcendental consciousness.

In recent years there has been an attempt to more carefully identify the subjective experience of transcendental consciousness, and to characterize this subjective experience by specific objective markers. The Transcendental Meditation technique is dynamic, having both an inward phase and an outward phase; during the 20 or so minutes of TM practice, subjects go in and out of transcendental consciousness many times.

Subjects report that in the inward phase, their mental activity settles down to quieter levels until they eventually transcend all mental activity, yet remain awake in the experience of transcendental consciousness. In the outward phase, they emerge from transcendental consciousness, and more excited states of mental activity gradually reappear, preparing the way to begin the inward phase again.

The degree of clarity of the experience of transcendental consciousness (subjectively reported) varies greatly, as do the frequency and duration of each of these inward and outward phases. Subjects who are overly tired before practicing Transcendental Meditation report having short periods of drowsiness or even sleep during meditation. Throughout the TM technique, there is often a mixture of the active waking state, drowsiness, sleep, relaxation, quiet waking state, and the experience of transcendental consciousness.

The mixture of states that occurs during TM practice is a direct consequence not only of the initial condition of the individual's nervous system, but also of the dynamics of the procedure itself. The deep rest during the technique allows the system to "normalize" itself—that is, to remove any functional or structural abnormalities and regain its normal healthy patterns of functioning. Everyone is familiar with this principle: when we rest during a cold or illness, the body's internal system spontaneously attempts to remove any foreign invaders and to heal itself.

The same principle applies to the practice of TM. As the mind becomes less active during TM, the body settles down and becomes restfully alert. Its internal systems automatically begin to remove any deep-seated stresses or abnormalities. This normalization process causes a stir of activity. The mind shifts out of transcendental consciousness, becoming more active as it returns to a more excited state, or becoming less active to the point of drowsiness or even sleep.

Several recent studies have used subjective reports coupled with certain objective criteria to help isolate and selectively study periods of transcendental consciousness. One of the important findings of these studies is that there are different physiological patterns of transcending for different individuals. For example, one study looked at the frequency of breath suspension in TM. This is a pattern often found in classical descriptions of the experience of transcending: a slowing or cessation of breathing and a sense of connectedness to the silence that upholds all nature. In the Vedic tradition the word *prana* has two distinct meanings: on the one hand, it refers to the most basic energy or primal force of the universe; on the other hand, it refers to individual breath. Likewise, the word *chi* in the Chinese tradition refers both to the primal energy of the universe and individual breath. And in the early Greek tradition, the word *pneuma* also has these two meanings.

In Transcendental Meditation, subjects sometimes describe their experience in terms of a momentary feeling that the breath has stopped and yet the body is filled with energy and pure awareness. Objective measurements of this experience do, in fact, show respiratory suspension for as much as one minute in about one-third of the TM subjects. When TM subjects are compared with nonmeditating controls who are simply resting with their eyes closed, it is found that the frequency, mean, maximum, and total episode lengths of these respiratory suspensions are all substantially greater in the TM group than in the controls. Further, when these TM subjects are instructed to push an event marker button after each experience of transcendental consciousness, an extremely large percentage of button presses occurs within a few seconds after the breath suspensions. Thus, for these subjects, periods of breath suspension can, in fact, be used as reliable physiological correlates of episodes of transcendental consciousness—they are an objective measure of the subjective patterns of transcendence.

Recent studies have extended these results and more carefully analyzed the neurophysiological control of respiratory patterns during the TM technique. These studies show both a decreased sensitivity to increased levels of carbon dioxide added to the air inhaled during meditation and an increased sensitivity to low levels of oxygen. This suggests an even more refined pattern of physiological functioning, indicating that there are specific alterations in centers within the brain that are involved with monitoring both carbon dioxide and oxygen levels.

What is perhaps most significant about these and other physiological studies is that they have shown us that transcending is not exclusively the province of Indian or even Eastern physiology. The machinery and patterns of transcending are part of the genetic endowment of the human nervous system. Whether we use it or not, transcending is an inherent ability. In fact, Western literature is filled with descriptions of states of restful alertness that are strikingly similar to the patterns of transcendental consciousness, as are the personal records of people in many different cultures throughout the ages. Although one rarely reads of anyone who regularly experienced this state via the use of a systematic technique, many have experienced it at least once or twice in their lives.

In "Tintern Abbey," Wordsworth vividly describes a transcendental experience that would be as comprehensible to a modern physiologist as to a Vedic sage:

> . . . that serene and blessed mood,
> In which the affections gently lead us on, —
> Until, the breath of this corporeal frame
> And even the motion of our human blood
> Almost suspended, we are laid asleep
> In body, and become a living soul:
> While with an eye made quiet by the power
> Of harmony and the deep power of joy,
> We see into the life of things.

Wordsworth describes his experience with great accuracy in these lines, specifically referring to both the suspension of breathing and changes in circulation—the same physiological patterns that our painstaking collection of scientific data on transcendental consciousness corroborates, more than 170 years later.

Patterns of the Brain

Conscious experience depends upon the proper functioning of our brain. One of the most frequently used objective measures to study the human brain and its relationship to consciousness is the electroencephalograph (EEG). EEG, which measures the patterns of brain wave activity, gives an overall measure of the electrical activity of specific regions of the brain.

EEG measurements have also been used to study meditation. My own early research on the Transcendental Meditation technique demonstrated increased activity in two types of EEG wave patterns: alpha waves, which have a frequency of about 8–10 cycles per second, and theta waves, 5–7 cycles per second. The changes reported were localized in the frontal parts of the brain.

The most commonly seen pattern was an increase in frontal theta waves and/or frontal slow alpha (8 cycles per second). These findings were replicated and extended by Dr. Jean-Paul Banquet and his co-workers at Massachusetts General Hospital. Dr. Banquet also found in certain subjects an increase in beta wave activity (20–40 cycles per second), associated with the subjective experience of transcending.

Another replication of these findings came from a study by Hebert and Lehman in Switzerland. The researchers noted that approximately one-third of the subjects practicing TM showed prominent high-voltage theta waves in the frontal areas of the brain. These theta waves took the form of spindles (a gradual increase and then a gradual diminution). The authors noted that these patterns were not found in the non-meditating control group.

Thus these combined studies document the emergence of four distinct EEG patterns during TM: (1) an increase in theta waves in frontal areas of the brain, (2) an increase in slow alpha waves, also in the frontal area, (3) an increase in frontal theta and slow alpha waves together, and (4) an increase in beta wave activity. Dr. Banquet suggested that these patterns were indicative of stages of transcending; however, more recent research by myself, Dr. Fred Travis, and Dr. David Orme-Johnson led me to conclude that they indicate individualized patterns of transcending, rather than specific stages. Further, recent research has revealed another interesting pattern—a shifting of the dominant alpha frequency either up or down by one or two cycles per second.

What is the basis of these patterns? Are there more patterns? Do they indicate styles of cognitive functioning that may be specific to each individual? I believe that by studying the functioning of the brain during transcending, when the mind is settling to its simplest state of awareness, we will be able to understand the fundamental modes of human intelligence and creativity. These questions suggest further avenues of inquiry that researchers including myself are currently pursuing.

EEG Coherence

One of the most important and useful developments in EEG research on TM has come through the application of a new measurement, EEG coherence. EEG coherence measures the *orderliness* of the electrical activity of the brain and helps answer the question, "Is the activity of one area of the brain correlated with the activity of another?" Measurements of coherence are derived from a sophisticated computer analysis of EEG signals, which compares the activity in two different regions of the brain and determines whether there is a stable relationship between them—that is, it indirectly measures their degree of integration.

Dr. Donald Walter, Dr. Ross Adey, and their co-workers at the UCLA Brain Research Institute were among the first to apply this measurement in studies distinguishing between states of awareness. For example, they noted a decrease in alpha and theta coherence during sleep. They speculated on the location of key brain centers that might be responsible for generating and synchronizing EEG signals. One of their most interesting findings occurred during the orbit of a Gemini spacecraft. During one 40-minute period, astronaut Frank Borman was very relaxed yet still awake. During that period his EEG coherence markedly increased in the theta frequency.

The first studies on EEG coherence during the Transcendental Meditation technique were conducted in 1976 and clearly showed an increase in alpha coherence during TM, with a spreading of EEG coherence to theta and beta frequencies. In a long-term meditator of 15 years, continuously strong coherence was seen concurrently in all EEG frequencies, both during and outside meditation. This was not observed in control subjects during either extended periods of eyes-closed relaxation or during "mock" meditations that involved nontaxing, repetitive backwards counting. In the mock meditation, alpha coherence tended to decrease throughout the period.

EEG coherence measurements during the TM technique helped further distinguish the pattern of physiological changes during TM from those seen in sleep or drowsiness; in both sleep and drowsiness any consistent, strong coherence in the alpha and theta bands is lost. Further, in TM subjects clearer experience of transcending was associated with higher levels of EEG coherence.

Later studies found a further pattern in some subjects: increased EEG alpha coherence in the frontal areas of the brain coupled with periods of respiratory suspension; and these were correlated with the subjective experience of transcendental consciousness. The EEG coherence of control subjects was measured while they voluntarily held their breaths, but there was no significant change during such periods. EEG coherence, especially when coupled with other measures such as respiration rate, thus proved to be a sensitive indicator of the experience of transcendental consciousness.

A further breakthrough in EEG research on TM came recently through the work of Dr. Nicolai Lyubimov, Director of the Neurocybernetics Laboratory at the Moscow Brain Research Institute. Dr. Lyubimov is one of the world's most distinguished neuroscientists, who became interested in conducting research on Transcendental Meditation several years ago in Russia.

His subsequent studies on long-term practitioners in Holland focused on a measure of EEG activity known as sensory evoked potentials, in which repeated sensory stimuli are given to subjects while the electrical response of the brain is simultaneously recorded. Sensory evoked potentials were recorded before, during, and after TM practice. Early components of the sensory evoked potential (those immediately following the stimulus) reflect basic mechanisms through which the brain begins to process incoming sensory data. Later components reflect more complex activity associated with learning, association, memory, emotion, and their interaction, as well as conscious awareness.

In the Holland studies, Dr. Lyubimov found that during Transcendental Meditation practice, early components of evoked potentials were distributed much more widely on the cerebral cortex than is usual, a pattern indicating that TM is a very dynamic process utilizing more areas of the brain than during normal waking activity. However, late components were diminished in both hemispheres, reflecting a reduction in complex processing and neural interaction, thus indicating a pattern associated with a simpler, quieter state of awareness.

Dr. Lyubimov feels that TM taps hidden reserves of the brain, electrical pathways that are not ordinarily in use. His previous research had demonstrated that after injury to the incoming (afferent) sensory fibers, the central nervous system can restore the flow of sensory information by mobilizing alternate central nervous system pathways of sensory input—in other words, hidden reserves. Dr. Lyubimov suggests that the changes in sensory evoked potentials during

Transcendental Meditation may be the physiological counterpart to the subjective experience of unbounded awareness.

These findings are important in that they give us a deeper understanding of the way we utilize the brain during Transcendental Meditation. They shed light on the mechanisms that may underlie and be responsible for the wide-ranging beneficial effects of the TM technique on cognitive functioning.

Patterns of Neurophysiological Development

Research on the Transcendental Meditation and TM-Sidhi program has identified not only the unique pattern of physiological changes during TM, but also an entire range of benefits in practically all areas of individual life, including health and aging. (We will discuss more about these benefits in later chapters.) Three recent studies have used a powerful advanced statistical technique known as *meta-analysis*.

The first meta-analysis, by Dr. Michael Dillbeck and Dr. Orme-Johnson, found significant differences on a number of variables between TM and ordinary rest, as well as showing that outside of meditation the TM subjects, compared to controls, had lower heart rates, respirations rates, and plasma lactate levels and greater stability of their autonomic nervous systems as indicated by basal skin resistance. This meta-analysis indicates that physiological and biochemical effects of TM carry over into activity.

A similar effect is seen in psychological studies. Dr. Kenneth Eppley and his co-workers published a meta-analysis study that examined over 100 studies on the effects on anxiety of many well-known meditation and relaxation techniques, including Transcendental Meditation and Progressive Muscle Relaxation. The researchers selected only the most well-designed research studies in which (a) the subjects were randomly chosen for the experimental and control group (this is known as random assignment), thus avoiding self-selection, and (b) there was a low drop-out rate. These selected studies had either been published in academic journals or published as doctoral dissertations. The results of this meta-analysis showed that TM was four times as effective in reducing anxiety as other techniques.

Finally, a third meta-analysis study, by Dr. Charles Alexander and his co-workers, found that, compared with other relaxation techniques,

Transcendental Meditation was substantially more effective in increasing self-actualization, a measure of psychological development.

From this and other research we can determine that the technologies of the Vedic paradigm are indeed the most effective in enabling us to transcend to the deeper layers of our subjective physiology and to unfold our full mental and physical potential.

These meta-analyses, as well as many psychological studies on the TM technique, have enabled researchers to objectively identify specific patterns of improvement at each level of our anatomy of consciousness. On the level of the ego, studies show increased self-actualization, enhanced self-concept and self-esteem, and enhanced self or ego development. On the level of the intellect, studies show increased intelligence, shorter choice reaction time, increased achievement on basic academic skills, and improved academic performance in higher education. On the level of the mind, there is increased creativity, increased efficiency of concept learning, broader comprehension, improved ability to focus attention, a more stable internal frame of reference, and improved memory, learning, and cognitive flexibility. On the level of the senses, studies show improved efficiency and flexibility of visual perception, increased field independence, shorter reaction time, and enhanced neuromuscular efficiency.

Thus the Vedic paradigm includes both an intellectual understanding of the anatomy of consciousness as well as a technology of consciousness to improve all its levels simultaneously. Further, it utilizes the tools of objective science, in the form of physiological and psychological measures, to verify these patterns in the unfoldment of human development. Maharishi's Vedic Science emphasizes that higher states of consciousness are natural; in higher states, we would expect that the physiology becomes much more integrated, complete, flexible, and balanced. These studies thus give us some idea of the direction of neurophysiological and psychological development as one grows towards higher states of consciousness.

Through Maharishi's technologies of consciousness, we now have the means for realizing the full range of human development—the state of enlightenment. Enlightenment as defined in the Vedic paradigm is not abstract or mystical—on the contrary, it is very practical, involving a holistic pattern of systematic refinement in neurophysiological functioning. The entire body of research has enabled us to establish, for the first time ever, the objective criteria for scientifically validating the development of higher states of consciousness.

THE CHEMISTRY
OF CONSCIOUSNESS

INDIA IS THE LAND OF MEDITATION, A LAND OF YOGIS AND
saints. Various forms of meditation are such an intimate part of
the tradition and culture that practically everyone is familiar with
it. When I once asked a bright young group of medical students
in South India whether they might be interested in meditation, especially if I could show strict scientific research on its benefits for learning, health, and longevity, very few expressed interest. I wasn't sure
whether this was because of the long-held misunderstanding that per-
vades India about the mystical and impractical nature of meditation, or
if it just came from the lack of a rational explanation for how something so familiar and common could have such good and scientifically
verifiable effects.

I then asked the students how many might be interested if I were to
offer a new pill, developed in our Western laboratories, which could
improve their memory and have beneficial effects on their health and
longevity. Virtually all the students raised their hands; they were more
than willing to take this new pill. Granted, these were medical students,
yet medical students are more aware than the public of the shortcom-
ings and side effects of pills. Why, then, were they so eager to take a
pill rather than meditate?

Finally I asked them that if I could demonstrate that during meditation a new chemical was produced, and that this chemical was identical to the pill I was offering them (i.e., it markedly improved mental and physical functioning), would they then be interested in meditation? This time the students all raised their hands enthusiastically.

As long as I could explain the mechanics of meditation in terms of pills and chemicals, then there was no prejudice, no misconception. Everyone takes pills for instant relief. We understand how they work, and we want even better ones. They are part of the classical paradigm. Meditation, however, is part of a new paradigm of consciousness. Only when meditation is explained in the mechanical terms of the old classical paradigm, does it become more readily acceptable.

Actually what I was offering to the students was not merely a fanciful idea. Today, laboratories around the world are attempting to isolate a single chemical that could help explain the physiological and psychological changes seen during the Transcendental Meditation and TM-Sidhi program—a single chemical that would link the physiology of consciousness with the physiology of matter.

Identifying Chemicals in the Brain

Several years ago, I had the opportunity to present a special award to Dr. Andrew Schally, a Nobel laureate. He was an extremely warm and friendly man of enormous energy and great accomplishment; at that time, he had over one thousand published papers. Before I met Dr. Schally, I had done some background reading to become more familiar with his research. I had come across a series of articles on a particular period in his career that resulted in his receiving the Nobel prize. Exciting and revealing, his story is indicative of the tremendous competition and progress over the last forty years in the field of brain chemistry, which has resulted in the discovery of numerous biochemicals that affect our health and behavior.

In the 1950s there was a firm belief that key substances produced by the brain controlled the actions of the master gland of the body, the pituitary. Two primary American laboratories were receiving considerable funds from the federal government to search for these special substances, referred to as "hypothalamic releasing factors." The hypothalamus is a tiny region of the brain that orchestrates many responses in the body, such as the "fight-or-flight" response that occurs in stressful situations. Both labs were looking for the hypothalamic releasing factor that controlled the production of the stress hormone ACTH from the pituitary. ACTH is produced during stress and, when released from the pituitary, causes the release of the hormone cortisol from the adrenal glands.

The two labs were racing with each other to isolate and identify this new powerful releasing factor, whose existence had been inferred from numerous experiments. To isolate and identify this substance was far from simple, consuming hundreds of thousands of dollars. Handling the substance required extreme measures because it could easily be broken down and destroyed. It was a Herculean task, which continued for several years.

Over time, other researchers became uneasy and even upset at the large sums of money being diverted to these projects. Did the substance really exist? At one point, the two key researchers, Dr. Schally and Dr. Guillemin, were asked to present their results. Neither one had firm evidence, but the Guillemin group had come across another new substance, also a hypothalamic releasing factor, that stimulated the pituitary gland to secrete a hormone that regulates the activity of the thyroid gland.

Unfortunately, the Guillemin group had only a small quantity of this new substance. While they could show its effects, Dr. Guillemin did not have enough to identify its complete structure. Nevertheless, because he needed to provide some evidence for the existence of hypothalamic releasing factors, he showed his results at a conference. The Schally group had also come across this same substance, but had not paid close attention to it. However, Schally's group had saved enough of the new substance so that once Dr. Guillemin's results were revealed, Dr. Schally could then analyze it and determine its precise structure.

In the end, both researchers shared the Nobel prize for their contribution to understanding and identifying hypothalamic releasing factors. Both groups went on to identify several more factors; however, for many years the ACTH releasing factor eluded them. Finally, the Guillemin group identified the structure of this substance. It had been a long and tiresome search; yet it has since inspired many other researchers and has demonstrated the importance of perseverance and commitment in uncovering nature's most precious secrets.

The same kind of difficult search has ensued for many new substances. And every year, more and more are identified. For example, as we mentioned earlier, several years ago scientists discovered the body's natural painkillers, the endorphins and enkephalins. These and other chemical communicators are the means by which impulses of thought, feeling, and perception—the fluctuations within the physiology of consciousness—manifest into the physiology of matter. Today the intense search continues, because these chemicals are believed to be the key to understanding and treating many diseases and abnormal behavior. Researchers know that if they can find one of these key new substances, a Nobel prize may well be within their grasp.

Ojas and Soma

Through the years Maharishi has referred many times to two substances frequently mentioned in the Vedic texts. These substances, known as *ojas* and *soma*, are considered to be the body's natural mediators of perfect health, longevity, and the experience of higher states of consciousness. Let's consider soma first.

Maharishi explains that in the Vedic literature, the word soma has several meanings. In its broadest sense, soma refers to a basic tendency of nature that holds the universe together, the flow of the underlying self-interacting dynamics of consciousness.

Soma also refers to a chemical produced in the body as a result of achieving a stress-free state of consciousness. As Maharishi describes,

> a normally functioning nervous system, free from stress and strain and any abnormality, produces a chemical called soma. . . . If there are no restrictions, no inhibitions, then awareness is unbounded, and when this unbounded awareness is maintained spontaneously at all times, then the nervous system is functioning normally. . . . Now the by-product of a normally functioning digestive system is soma. Soma is that which helps all the fundamentals of individual life to develop themselves so that the totality of individual consciousness may rise above boundaries, and have an unbounded status.

In this context, soma is both the product of neurophysiological refinement and the very substance that enables the development of full mental and physical potential. The principle that every state of consciousness is supported by a physiological state is interpreted here to mean that soma is the key biochemical that supports the experience of transcendental consciousness and eventually enlightenment. This "elixir of longevity" is distilled not in a pharmaceutical lab, but through the process of the inner development of consciousness. Soma is a product of the body's natural pharmacy, created by a nervous system functioning in higher states of consciousness.

Certain texts in the Vedic literature that pertain specifically to health further elaborate the definition of soma. In these, "soma" refers specifically to the first definition—an abstract dynamical principle of consciousness that is capable of unifying diversity in nature. For the second definition (a unique chemical in the body responsible for ideal health and longevity), the term ojas is used. Ojas and soma are intimately related. They represent the same unifying principle in nature. However, soma is that unmanifest principle expressed in consciousness; ojas is its manifest expression as the finest possible level of matter. We could say that ojas is the first material, biochemical expression of soma in the physiology of matter, which is the basis of all the succeeding layers of matter in the body—cells, tissues, organs, etc.

Ojas is considered a biochemical that establishes balance between the physiology of consciousness and the physiology of matter. Because it is located at the junction point between consciousness and matter, ojas is described as being like "a lamp at the door," illuminating both the inner field of consciousness and the outer field of matter.

One last definition of soma: the Vedic literature also refers to a particular plant or herb of this name, traditionally used during special ceremonies. Among the many medicinal properties attributed to this plant is the ability to increase longevity. In the context of the previous discussion, we could understand this definition of soma as yet another aspect—a more concrete, manifest expression—of its nature as the self-interacting dynamics of consciousness, which supports and promotes the evolution of everything.

Searching for the Biochemical Basis of Transcendental Consciousness

For several years, researchers have been trying to better understand the neurophysiological and biochemical mechanisms of Transcendental Meditation. They have, in fact, been involved in a search for ojas and soma. One of the most active research groups, at the University of California at Irvine, has made significant contributions in the search for a biochemical understanding of meditation during the last 15 years.

Their initial studies compared important hormones and basic amino acids in the blood of meditating individuals with those of resting controls. Further, they were able to map specific changes in blood flow to the various organs of the body.

Their studies concluded that Transcendental Meditation produces an integrated response that involves coordinated physiological changes different from those found in dreaming, drowsiness, and deep sleep. For example, they found that during and after meditation, the stress hormone cortisol decreases. They also reported an increase in levels of the amino acid phenylalanine, which suggests changes in the metabolism of the key brain neurotransmitters, the catecholamines. Finally, they investigated a pituitary hormone known as antidiuretic hormone, or ADH. This hormone, in addition to its effects on water regulation, has been associated with improved memory. Meditators were found to have unusually high levels of this hormone. (This substantiates other findings that TM improves memory and recall.)

The greater part of their research, however, has focused on identifying a possible new factor produced in the blood that might be responsible for metabolic changes. In earlier studies my co-workers and I had found that a chemical called lactic acid, or lactate, decreased markedly during TM. Lactate is a by-product of *anaerobic* metabolism in cells, which does not involve oxygen. This process is less efficient than the normal *aerobic* metabolism, which uses oxygen and eliminates carbon dioxide. In an extensive study, the Irvine group found significantly decreased levels of lactic acid production in isolated red blood cells from meditators as compared with nonmeditating controls. Since nothing else is known to cause such an effect, they postulated the existence of some new factor in the blood that would be capable of improving metabolic efficiency.

Most recently they have found changes in oxygen and carbon dioxide levels in the blood, suggesting a marked alteration in basic metabolic and biochemical pathways. The ratio of carbon dioxide eliminated to oxygen consumed (known as the respiratory quotient) in the cells of the forearm is usually 0.8, or at the lowest 0.6; however, during the TM technique this ratio decreases to near zero. This suggests that during TM the body may switch to other biochemical pathways that do not produce carbon dioxide, or that utilize it in a different way. In order for the metabolism to switch to these pathways, it is likely that different key biochemicals such as enzymes might be produced during TM. The investigation of these specialized metabolic pathways thus might lead to the discovery of previously unknown chemical factors that are produced during the TM technique.

Long-Term Hormonal Changes with the TM-Sidhi Program

In Switzerland a research group looked at changes in hormones over several years in subjects practicing the Transcendental Meditation and TM-Sidhi program. Blood samples were taken before subjects were instructed in the advanced TM-Sidhi program and then once each year for the next three years. The blood samples were analyzed for several chemical factors, including important pituitary hormones. The pituitary gland, as I mentioned earlier, is the master gland of the body, and the hormones it secretes often regulate the activity of the other glands. For example, the pituitary gland secretes a hormone known as thyroid-stimulating hormone, or TSH, that directly influences the activity of the thyroid gland. When TSH levels increase, thyroid hormone levels increase; when TSH levels decrease, thyroid hormone levels decrease.

In the study, TSH in people practicing the TM-Sidhi program decreased markedly over three years with little or no decrease in the thyroid hormones. This unusual result suggests a significant increase in the sensitivity of the thyroid gland's receptors as the result of the TM-Sidhi program.

These findings are interesting in light of other research findings. With age, levels of TSH usually become elevated, presumably due to the decreased sensitivity of the thyroid gland. The proposed increased thyroid sensitivity caused by the TM-Sidhi program may be an indication of a more youthful and optimal state of physiological functioning.

The changes seen in the TM and TM-Sidhi program may also be due to changes in another important gland—the pineal gland. For many years no one knew the role of this pine cone–shaped gland, which sits at the center of the brain. We now know that it plays an important regulatory role in biological rhythms and hormonal activity. The gland itself is sensitive to cycles of light and dark and secretes melatonin, a hormone that has many effects throughout the body. The decrease in TSH and the changes in two other pituitary hormones (growth hormone and prolactin), which are also reported to occur as a result of the TM-Sidhi program, could be a result of increased melatonin production. Research is in progress to determine if the pineal hormone melatonin is in fact the biochemical basis of the changes during Transcendental Meditation, or is related to them.

Is the Biochemical Basis of Transcending a Neurotransmitter?

Another approach several groups in Europe and the United States have taken to find the biochemical basis of Transcendental Meditation is to investigate neurotransmitters. Neurotransmitters are chemical substances released when one nerve cell wants to communicate with another. Messages in the brain are transmitted electrically along nerve fibers. However, when nerve fibers of different cells come together, there is a tiny gap, the synapse, that separates them. For the message to travel from one nerve fiber to another, it must bridge the synapse through the release of one or more neurotransmitters.

Imbalance in the brain's neurotransmitters is believed to be the cause of some physical and mental diseases. For example, low levels of the neurotransmitter dopamine in a certain area of the brain are consistently found in patients with Parkinson's disease. Most modern treatments of this disease involve the intake of substances that increase dopamine. The neurotransmitter serotonin has been implicated in many behavioral states. Low levels are associated with increased incidence of depression, suicide, and aggression.

Several years ago, a research group led by Dr. Bujatti at the University of Vienna analyzed serotonin levels during the TM technique. The researchers indirectly measured serotonin levels by measuring its by-products in the urine. Within the body, chemical substances such as neurotransmitters are continually being made and broken down. Once broken down, they are eliminated in the urine. The main by-product of serotonin is called 5-hydroxyindoleacetic acid (5-HIAA). Since serotonin is produced not only in the brain but also in other parts of the body, the levels of 5-HIAA reflect overall serotonin metabolism. The study compared urine samples of 5-HIAA taken before and after meditation with those taken before and after rest in control subjects.

The most interesting results showed that the meditators had higher resting levels of 5-HIAA than controls. These levels increased significantly after meditation but not after rest in the control subjects. Dr. Bujatti speculated that the activity of the neurotransmitter serotonin increases during TM, and that just as adrenaline plays an important role in orchestrating the physiological changes of the fight-or-flight response, serotonin plays an important role in the physiological changes of a "rest-and-fulfillment" response during TM.

Several other researchers, such as Dr. Ken Walton, a neurochemist at Maharishi International University, also feel that serotonin is involved in the biochemical basis of transcending. Dr. Walton and his co-workers have conducted a number of studies. Most recently they have found that TM meditators as compared to controls have lower resting levels of the stress hormone cortisol and high levels of a hormone known as dehydroepiandrosterone, which is associated with better health (we will learn more about this hormone in Chapter 8). Dr. Walton suggests that these beneficial hormonal changes are related in turn to changes in serotonin activity in the brain, which occur as a result of the TM technique.

The Mind-Body Network

The search for the biochemical basis of transcending is one of the most exciting frontiers in research on the Vedic paradigm. It is part of a new attempt in science to uncover the biochemical basis of subjective states of consciousness. The great value of such research is that it will establish a bridge between the divergent understandings of the physiology of consciousness and the physiology of matter.

We are beginning to think of the body not as a localized bundle of cells and tissues, but as one mind-body network of intelligence. The primary means for the integration of this mind-body network is through chemical communicators such as hormones, neurotransmitters, and neuropeptides. Recent discoveries about the action of neuropeptides in mediating behavior have given us a far more detailed understanding of how this mind-body network functions. These discoveries have been enriched by the finding that many different types of cells throughout the body can both send and receive messages via the neuropeptides. As more and more biochemical messengers are discovered, the picture will become increasingly more comprehensive.

Integrating modern scientific discovery of the mind-body network with the ancient understanding and technologies of the Vedic paradigm will give us the means to thoroughly examine the physiology of consciousness. We will be able to objectively discern the fine details of the mind-body network. Further, as a result of this integrated research, we will finally have a complete system of knowledge, understandable to scientist and layperson alike, of the underlying biochemical mechanics of the development of higher states of consciousness.

CHAPTER 4

CONSCIOUSNESS
AND HEALTH

A
COUPLE OF YEARS AGO I HAD AN APPOINTMENT TO MEET
with a fellow researcher at a prestigious New York hospital. When I arrived, I was invited to wait in the head cardiologist's office. As I entered the room I noticed a live
video monitor connected to the main operating room, on which I
could hear and see an open-heart surgery actually taking place.

A very angry surgeon was interrogating the cardiologist about his
diagnosis. The patient's chest lay open, but the surgeon could find
nothing wrong with the heart! The cardiologist maintained that all the
preoperative tests had shown that one of the heart valves was malfunctioning. The surgeon could see that this was simply not so. Everything
was perfectly normal. The discussion went on; the patient, his chest
open, lay unconscious on the table between them. Finally, in an aggressive tone, the surgeon said, "Well now that I'm in here, I'm going to
replace the valve anyway!"

I had lived most of my life with great confidence in modern medicine. How naive was I? Should I blame the cardiologist or the surgeon?
I knew enough about biomedical equipment to know how difficult it
can be to interpret certain results. I also knew that what I had witnessed was not exactly an everyday occurrence. Yet I was, and still am

appalled at a system that is so complex and out of the patient's grasp that we can become the victims not only of disease but also of its treatment. Even with the most sophisticated tools and years of medical training, it is not only possible, but not uncommon, for doctors and even specialists to incorrectly diagnose and treat a critical condition. Iatrogenic disease, the disorders caused by modern medicine, is widespread and of grave concern today.

Just entering a hospital can be a risky act. For example, as reported in the *New England Journal of Medicine*, researchers studied the course of medication prescribed to 816 people admitted consecutively by a hospital. Of these patients, 36% suffered adverse side effects of their medication. Another study followed 3,181 children who visited a general pediatrics group practice during the course of one year. More than 30% of the children experienced one or more adverse drug reactions. This is also commonly seen in the elderly, who are most easily harmed by the prescription of multiple drugs with potentially fatal interactions. As the title of an editorial in *The Lancet* asked, "Need we poison the elderly so often?"

Surveys show that 89% of the American population is dissatisfied with modern medicine and recognizes the need for major changes. While the inadequacies and rising costs of modern medicine cause serious problems in the U.S., they cause almost insurmountable ones in most developing countries.

Next to improved hygiene, the single most important breakthrough in medical history has probably been the discovery of antibiotics. But because of widespread and often excessive use of antibiotics, many viruses and bacteria have altered their genetic codes and have become increasingly more resistant and deadly. The worst of these new strains of bacteria reside in hospitals where antibiotics are most frequently used. Hospital-acquired infections from these bacteria are becoming increasingly more prevalent.

Perhaps the most surprising inadequacy of modern medicine is its inability to prevent the two greatest killers today, heart disease and cancer. Despite the vast amounts of money spent on research and medical care, these two diseases are still the greatest threats to our lives. At present rates, one out of every two people in America alive today will die of heart disease, and one out of four will die of cancer.

We often hear a great deal about the progress made by modern medicine in saving the lives of patients with heart disease; however, when we examine the actual data, it is not so obvious. For example, the typical "improvement" over one year in the number of lives lost due to heart disease for a population of 100,000 people is only three. That means for a town of the size of Santa Fe, only three fewer people than the year before died of heart disease.

The war against cancer is a complicated issue. A study published in the *New England Journal of Medicine* found that for the majority of cancers there has been no real progress over the past three decades in terms of mortality rates, despite millions of dollars spent on research and the widespread use of costly and highly toxic treatments. According to the authors, "We are losing the war against cancer."

The problem is the enormous emphasis we put on treating the symptoms of disease and how little we do to prevent them. For example, the most popular operation for treating heart disease in the United States is coronary bypass surgery. The coronary arteries are the vessels that feed oxygen to the heart muscle. When they become clogged with fat deposits, there is a great chance for a heart attack. During surgery the clogged arteries are bypassed by splicing in a piece of vein from the leg, thus providing an alternate route for the flow of blood. When bypass surgery was first performed in the late sixties, it was hailed as the pinnacle of success in modern medicine. Patients reported an immediate relief of symptoms. They were able to move about without the previous constant pain. Operations were performed for many years without any serious scientific evaluation.

When coronary bypass surgery was finally evaluated in several major studies, it was shown that overall it did not change the course of the disease nor even prolong the life of the individual when compared with conventional drug therapy. The new vessels can become clogged as soon as two years after the operation. To be fair, there are two special cases when this operation does seem to have some beneficial value. But these cases do not account for the staggering number of operations performed each year—approximately 300,000.

Why is this? Doctors feel obligated both legally and morally to offer their patients the best of modern medical technologies, and patients often would rather have immediate relief, even if the long-term prognosis isn't as reassuring. In the future, coronary bypass surgery most likely will be replaced by new technologies. It is hoped that these procedures will be less invasive, but will they be any better? No one knows yet. As was the case with coronary bypass surgery, it may be years before they are properly evaluated.

The Damaging Effects of Stress

In the 14th century, an epidemic of plague wiped out one-third of Europe's population in less than one hundred years. The epidemic of the modern world is stress. Heart disease is the number one stress-related disorder and is by far the greatest health problem of the Western world. It causes more adult deaths than all other diseases combined.

While there are clearly genetic factors (and others such as diet and smoking) that make some individuals more predisposed to heart disease, it is stress that ultimately precipitates the fatal attack. Stress is a hidden killer; it is all around us and continually affects our physiologies.

There are numerous factors known to increase stress, including the death of a loved one, loss of a job, financial difficulties, divorce, lack of sleep, and tense work situations. One stress seems to attract another, and the cumulative action of multiple stresses has even more damaging effects on the body. Stress disrupts the flow of intelligence in our physiology of consciousness; it manifests as structural or functional abnormalities deposited in the system and eventually results in disease in our physiology of matter.

To a large extent, the current understanding of the physiological manifestations of stress comes from the work of the late Dr. Hans Selye. He observed the reaction of animals to an overload of stress and defined three stages that form the basis of what he called the General Adaptation Syndrome. The three stages are: (1) the alarm reaction, (2) resistance, and (3) exhaustion.

The initial alarm reaction, sometimes referred to as the "fight-or-flight" response described in the previous chapter, is triggered by certain centers in the brain and results in a wide variety of changes throughout the body, including increased adrenaline levels in the blood, increased heart rate, elevation of blood sugar, and an entire redistribution of blood flow to ensure adequate supply to the brain, heart, and muscles.

In prolonged stress, the animal enters the second phase of the

General Adaptation Syndrome, resistance, in which the reactions of the nervous system and endocrine system seem to decrease, as if the animal has successfully adapted to the stressor. This is, however, not the case. The effects of stress are continually sapping the strength of the animal's physiology; the fight-or-flight response has merely diminished, just as the light from a flashlight grows dimmer from constant use. The unremitting stress leads to the third and terminal stage—exhaustion. In this stage the symptoms of the first stage reappear with much greater severity, and the animal dies if untreated.

Selye also found that if, during the stage of resistance, a second stress confronts the animal, the entire adaptive mechanism breaks down more easily, and the exhaustion stage rapidly sets in. Many diseases such as ulcers, insomnia, and headaches are thought to be due in part, or at least complicated by, an inappropriate or prolonged response to multiple-stress situations. Each day, whether caused by a traffic jam, a boss's remark, or a quarrel at home, the harmful effects of the stress response are having an impact on our health and longevity. It is no wonder that the harmful effects of stress are so strongly linked to heart disease.

Until very recently, heart attacks and strokes were considered a by-product of aging. Scientists have observed for many decades that blood vessels become narrow and less flexible with aging. Also, the buildup of hard, fatty deposits inside the artery walls increases year by year in many people, leading to high blood pressure, heart attacks, and strokes. The majority of Americans show these conditions as they age. However, more and more studies suggest that this process is neither normal nor inevitable. It is a product of our stressful civilization and of our inability to deal with the increasingly fast pace of life.

There are some simple cultures, removed from the stresses of Western life, which have almost no heart disease. This is the good news. We don't all have to be subjected to the newest operations of modern medicine. If nature did not mean for the heart and arteries to degenerate with age, then heart conditions should be preventable and reversible if caught in time. Recent research indicates that this is indeed possible. Dr. Dean Ornish, a San Francisco cardiologist, reported that 40 patients with advanced heart disease unblocked their coronary arteries through simple yoga exercises, meditation, and a strict low-cholesterol diet.

Evolution Management

Rest and relaxation can help relieve some symptoms of cardiovascular disease. Patients forced by their doctors to go to the hospital often temporarily recover from the adverse symptoms of cardiovascular disease just because they are forced to rest. Yet it is almost impossible in this day and age to have prolonged rest. Therefore, the only practical approach is to try to periodically quiet down and relax our overactive systems. That's why stress management programs have become very popular in the last ten years. There are many programs, and almost all of them work on the principle of relaxation. If stress arouses the physiology, then the way to counteract stress is to "de-arouse" the physiology—to relax.

Rest and relaxation can be antidotes to stress. Sleep itself removes stress. But usually the rest and relaxation of normal sleep is not enough, and sometimes we are actually too stressed to sleep. Stress management programs offer some small help by periodically reducing our level of stress. Occasional relaxation during the day can counter a few of the adverse effects of stress and fatigue. However, most stress management programs offer only superficial rest and relaxation. We need a far deeper rest to remove the deep-seated stresses that accumulate in our lives. These deep-seated stresses create subtle imbalances in our physiology, which, when they accumulate, lead to disease.

Where does stress enter the body? It enters through consciousness. Before a stressful experience affects our body it must usually first pass through our senses and emotions to the central nervous system. The brain acts as a filtering device that sorts which experiences are to be recorded and responded to. Filtering enables us to cope with all the external demands of the environment. If this coping ability is somehow hampered or overburdened, then stresses freely accumulate and tax our entire body.

How do we increase our coping ability? According to Maharishi, the key to managing stress is to transcend and evolve to higher states of consciousness. If we want to remove darkness from a room, we don't try to manage the darkness. Darkness is merely the absence of light. By turning on a light switch we automatically remove the darkness. Likewise, the way to remove stress is to go beyond it, to evolve. The process of transcending in Transcendental Meditation takes the mind to the state of pure consciousness, which is entirely free from stress. Unlike sleep or relaxation, in which the body is resting but the mind is either unconscious or dull, transcendental consciousness is a state in which the body is resting deeply while the mind is filled with unbounded awareness and bliss. It is a type of rest in which the nervous system becomes highly integrated and coherent. This restful alertness is not only the most powerful antidote to stress, but the most effective way to remove deep-rooted stresses already deposited in our nervous system.

Further, the regular experience of transcending acquaints the nervous system, little by little, with a state in which silence and activity can coexist. As we develop towards cosmic consciousness, we can be immersed in rigorous activity, yet not lose the experience of unbounded awareness. We are no longer overshadowed or exhausted by stressful experiences and therefore are better able to cope with environmental stress. As described in Chapter 1, experiences no longer leave deep impressions etched in our nervous system; the impression is more like a line on water. Many studies on the Transcendental Meditation and TM-Sidhi program show precisely this effect. When TM and TM-Sidhi subjects were given stressful stimuli, they were physiologically able to recover far more quickly than nonmeditating controls. The meditators also showed many long-term physiological and biochemical changes, indicating improved neurophysiological functioning.

The Transcendental Meditation and TM-Sidhi program enables individuals to evolve to healthier states. The TM technique has often been referred to as a "stress management" technique. It is indeed a powerful technique for the management of stress—but that is merely one of its positive side effects. The primary purpose of the technique is "evolution management," the development of higher states of consciousness, so that we can begin to use the full potential of the nervous system and live in perfect health.

Improving Cardiovascular Risk Factors

Over the past twenty years many scientific studies have confirmed the beneficial effects of the Transcendental Meditation and TM-Sidhi program on major cardiovascular risk factors. Independent studies at major medical schools have shown repeatedly that TM significantly reduces both systolic and diastolic blood pressure, particularly in patients who have recently developed high blood pressure. Several other studies have also shown that the TM technique is not only a curative for high blood pressure, but a preventive as well. Even elderly TM practitioners have lower blood pressures in general than nonmeditators. For example, TM subjects over the age of 50 had blood pressures lower than those of the average 30-year-old. On the whole, the longer people practice TM, the lower their blood pressure.

The most recent and well-controlled study, led by Dr. Robert Schneider and his co-workers, investigated the effects of TM on approximately 130 African Americans living in an urban setting. Subjects were randomly assigned to one of two experimental groups, a TM or a Progressive Muscle Relaxation (PMR) group, or to a "usual-care" control group. The usual-care control subjects received instructions for weight loss, salt restriction, alcohol moderation, and exercise. The experimental groups were carefully matched for factors that might influence the outcome, such as expectation of results, expertise and motivation of instructor, amount of time involved in instruction, and time involved in daily home practice. Both groups had about 90% compliance. About one-half the subjects were taking antihypertension medication; their doses were kept constant throughout the study. After three months, the TM group showed significantly greater reduction in both systolic and diastolic blood pressure, compared to the PMR group and the control group. The study is now being expanded and extended over a longer period, having received a major grant from the National Institutes of Health.

Researchers have also investigated the effects of the TM technique on high cholesterol. In one study, patients with high levels of cholesterol were divided into two groups, one that started the TM technique and a nonmeditating control group matched for age, gender, diet, weight, and initial cholesterol values. After one year the meditators' cholesterol levels had dropped significantly, while the controls' levels had not changed. In another study by the same researchers, subjects with normal cholesterol levels showed significant decreases in both cholesterol and blood pressure after practicing TM for six months as compared with controls.

Several studies have also demonstrated the positive effects of the

TM program on two other cardiovascular risk factors—smoking and obesity. In a large study of almost 2,000 people, subjects reported a significant reduction in cigarette smoking after starting TM. In another study, researchers surveyed a group of college students and older TM participants and found that overweight subjects tended to lose weight and underweight subjects tended to gain weight.

A recent study also examined the effects of Transcendental Meditation on individuals with certain personality traits. The hostility component of "Type A" behavior has been correlated with the greater occurrence and prevalence of coronary heart disease. The hostile Type A person is typically the busy, stressed professional who is relatively easily provoked into outbursts of anger and aggression. The results of the study suggested that TM beneficially modified the physiological and hormonal responses in these individuals, giving them a response pattern that was more similar to healthier Type B subjects. The study also showed that meditators exhibited an adaptive response known as "reduced end organ sensitivity." End organ sensitivity refers to the way in which cell receptors respond to stress hormones and neurotransmitters. The sensitivity of important cardiovascular receptors (β-adrenergic receptors) was shown to be reduced in meditators, thus enabling them to better adapt to the excessive physiological effects of stress.

Another clinical study looked at patients with angina pectoris. Those who began TM showed a marked improvement in their physiological responses to exercise compared with the nonmeditating controls. These and other studies suggest that the TM technique has an important effect in preventing and improving heart disease.

A Breakthrough Study on Health Insurance

To date, one of the most important health-related studies on the effects of the Transcendental Meditation and TM-Sidhi program is one which examined the statistics of a worldwide, highly respected health insurance company over a five-year period. The study compared several groups of professionals with a group of 2,000 members participating in the TM program. All the groups had health insurance with this same company. The study controlled for many factors that might affect health care use, such as age, gender, profession, cost-sharing, and geographic distribution. None of these factors could account for the meditators' dramatically lower insurance usage.

The TM group had consistently lower rates of hospitalization and doctor visits than the average of all other groups. In every category of disease, the medical care utilization of the TM group was considerably less than that of the industry norms. In most cases the differences were striking. For example, health care costs related to heart disease were 87% lower than the norm for the TM group. The rate of hospital admission for the TM group was 63% lower than the norm for non-surgical medical procedures, and 71.5% lower for surgery. The rate of doctor visits was 58.8% lower. These differences were not due to meditators intentionally avoiding medical care—for example, health care usage rates for obstetrics were similar in both groups.

One of the most significant findings was that the decrease in health care utilization was even more striking for older people. Meditators over 40 showed health care costs that were, on average, 75% lower than those for nonmeditators in the same age group. This would seem to indicate that the beneficial effects of the TM program actually increase as we get older. As a result of this study, one large insurance company in Europe reduced rates for TM practitioners by 30%. By using an effective evolution management program, we have the potential to prevent and even reverse many health disorders, including (as we will explore more fully in Chapter 8) the negative effects of aging.

A more recent longitudinal study evaluated the impact of TM on medical costs in French Canadians. The study controlled for age, gender, inflation (physicians' fees index), year-specific variation, and season, and adjusted expenses were analyzed three years before and after subjects started the TM technique. During the pretest the TM subjects' average expenses were not significantly different from the average of all enrollees in the Quebec health plan of the same age and gender. During posttest, the TM subjects' expenses declined 12% annually. The sample was subdivided to evaluate those who incurred the highest costs in the pre-TM period regardless of age. During posttest, high-cost cases declined even more than the others did— 18% annually. The expenses for subjects 50–82 years old were also evaluated and found to decline 19% annually. These results confirm and extend the earlier study.

These studies have extremely important implications for our own health care system as well as those of other nations. Health care in the United States is in the midst of a losing battle. Costs are increasing at an alarming rate. From 1970 to 1992, medical costs in the U.S. soared from $75 billion to $800 billion. This represents more than 13 percent of the gross national product. In addition, 50 million Americans have inadequate health insurance, and 37 million people have no insurance at all. Everyone agrees that something must be done, but no one has a solution.

The problem is even more devastating for developing nations, where there is a pressing need to update diagnostic and therapeutic medical equipment. The costs are so astronomical that such equipment is either nonexistent or in very limited supply. How do we resolve this growing dilemma? The only tenable answer is prevention. We must shift our emphasis to a prevention-oriented health care system.

The studies on the TM technique give us the answer as to how we can immediately and dramatically reduce health care costs. The reduction in health care costs found with meditators is extremely promising and gives clear evidence of the value of this preventive approach. Some may argue that more and larger studies are needed. There is no question that it would be ideal to study the effect of the TM program on larger populations. But at a time when many nations face spiraling medical costs, we must introduce simple and effective time-tested measures today; the most powerful and most extensively studied measure is the Transcendental Meditation technique.

Maharishi Ayur-Ved

Just as modern science has its practical application in modern medicine, Maharishi's Vedic Science and Technology has its practical application in a health care system known as Maharishi Ayur-Ved.

Ayur-Ved, one branch of the timeless tradition of Vedic wisdom, is the world's most comprehensive system of natural health care. The term Ayur-Ved comes from two Sanskrit words, *ayus*, meaning "life" or "lifespan," and *Ved*, meaning "knowledge" or "science." Ayur-Ved may be translated as "the science of life" or, more specifically, "the science of lifespan." Ayur-Ved includes knowledge about every aspect of life and health. However, particularly due to India's history of political turbulence, over hundreds of years, this knowledge became fragmented;

much of it was forgotten, and the rest was known to just a few experts.

In the 1980s, the complete and holistic value of Ayur-Ved was brought to light by Maharishi from the Vedic literature as part of his revitalization of the ancient Vedic wisdom. One of his first contributions to Ayur-Ved was the restoration of mental techniques, such as TM, to unfold the full potential of the physiology of consciousness. Originally these were an integral part of Ayur-Ved, but they had become de-emphasized or abandoned. Maharishi's next step was to work with the leading remaining experts of traditional Ayur-Ved to restore the completeness of this knowledge.

Once this complete and authentic system, known as Maharishi Ayur-Ved, had been formulated, lectures and symposia were held at leading research institutes and universities around the world to encourage scientific research on all the various therapeutic strategies of Maharishi Ayur-Ved. In the United States, experts in Maharishi Ayur-Ved spoke to such prominent forums as the National Institutes of Health, Johns Hopkins Medical School, Yale Medical School, Harvard School of Public Health, and Massachusetts General Hospital. Everywhere, they were received with great interest, and many studies have since been undertaken to investigate the programs of Maharishi Ayur-Ved.

Today, few people think of India as a source for new knowledge about health. There is no question that India has severe health problems. More than any other country, it needs a prevention-oriented approach, starting with the teaching of basic personal hygiene in the villages and extending to introduction of the complete approaches of Maharishi Ayur-Ved to help prevent the alarming rate of new incidence of disease, especially in urban areas.

To overcome our prejudices, we must understand that just because Transcendental Meditation and Maharishi's Vedic Science come from India, that doesn't make their application specific to that culture. The fact that Einstein, a German Jew, arrived at his famous theory of relativity while working at a patent office in Switzerland doesn't make his theory Swiss, German, or Jewish. In our age of science we are able to perceive principles of nature that transcend cultural boundaries and traditions. The Vedic paradigm is derived from universal principles of nature governing the dynamics of consciousness. The technologies of the Vedic paradigm, including the TM technique, reveal to us the inherent ability of our nervous system to experience those dynamics of consciousness and unfold our full mental and physical potential.

The entire world is in great need of a new medicine, one which encompasses both the modern technology of our age and the ancient understanding and technologies of the Vedic paradigm. Only by shifting our attention away from a totally disease-oriented approach and by recognizing the need for a preventive approach with a profound basis in knowledge and effective practices, will we be able to curb increasing health care costs. Only by better understanding the fundamental principles that govern our physiology of consciousness, as well as our physiology of matter, will we be able to eliminate today's major killer-diseases and promote an ideal state of health for every person in the world.

PART 2

THE PHYSIOLOGY
OF MATTER

CHAPTER 5

THE FINEST LAYERS OF OUR PHYSIOLOGY OF MATTER

S EVERAL YEARS AGO I ESCORTED A DISTINGUISHED PHYSICIAN and scientist—a woman responsible for the health care of several million people in her own country—through one of the first Maharishi Ayur-Ved clinics in North America. After touring the facility she sat in on several interviews with patients. The first case she heard was that of a young woman named Anne, age thirty-two. Anne was having a regular checkup and reported some sleep disorders and indigestion.

After a physical examination that involved both a routine Western and more specialized Ayurvedic examination, the clinic's doctor told her that she had been experiencing some unusual anger for the last three days. Now, Anne had been perfectly calm throughout, with no physiological or psychological evidence of anger. She was visibly surprised and said, "Yes, I have been angry at several things lately. How did you know? Did my husband tell you?" "No," the doctor laughed, "no one told me. It is one of the primary symptoms of your particular body type when there is a metabolic imbalance, and this imbalance is quite evident from your examination. I'm going to prescribe a few simple changes in diet and daily routine which will correct it."

After Anne had left the room, our visitor turned to the doctor in amazement. "How could you possibly determine that this lady has been angry for three days?" He explained that Anne's particular body type was prone to the emotion of anger, and also that Anne's responses to a diagnostic questionnaire and her pulse diagnosis gave clear indications of certain imbalances. The visitor witnessed several such displays of diagnosis, and by the end of the visit she was both impressed and enthusiastic. I had no difficulty explaining the concept of Ayurvedic body typing and its great value in helping to cure and, more importantly, prevent disease.

The Fundamental Structure of Matter

Maharishi Ayur-Ved, as we have described, is Maharishi's restoration of India's timeless health care system—the grandfather of natural medical systems. Maharishi Ayur-Ved contains highly refined techniques for both the diagnosis and treatment of disease. These techniques are based on an understanding of the physiology of consciousness and the physiology of matter that sees the body as an integrated whole, a network of intelligence, which is the microcosm of all of nature. The physician can enter this network through various means.

One of the central concepts described in classical Ayurvedic texts is known as Panchamahabhuta. This describes how matter arises from consciousness. What is particularly interesting in this theory is the description of the finer layers of our physiology of matter.

In this theory, the universe's origin is *avyakt*, "unmanifest"—the unmanifest unified field of pure consciousness. Arising from this field (the Self) are the various levels of the physiology of consciousness described earlier: ego, intellect, mind, and senses. As we pointed out in Chapter 1, these levels form the "anatomy" of consciousness. They are broad principles and structures of natural law at the foundation of everything in creation—the basis for the physiology of matter of the entire universe, which includes the human body.

As the laws of nature sequentially unfold through the self-interacting dynamics of pure consciousness, Maharishi explains how eventually the structures of natural law take on a concrete form, and consciousness gives rise to matter:

Through sequential development consciousness unfolds itself into the value of matter; consciousness becomes matter. The Self becomes

70

mind, and mind becomes matter. We see this in modern physiology, when the DNA and RNA give rise to all the proteins, which in turn structure the body systems. This transformation of the field of pure knowledge rising from DNA as the impulse of information in RNA, to RNA becoming protein and protein becoming the whole material system is the description of consciousness becoming matter.

There is thus a transition point in the sequential unfoldment of natural law, at which the subjective physiology of consciousness gives rise to the objective physiology of matter. Maharishi explains that this, too, is a self-referral process. He describes how this intimate and delicate connection between consciousness and matter takes place at the point when the subjective impulse of thought is becoming translated, through the DNA (deoxyribonucleic acid), into RNA (ribonucleic acid) and then into proteins, including neuropeptides, that comprise the biochemistry of thought:

> This transformation is sequential but always self-referral. It is like the airplane flying but always remaining self-referral to the ground station through the radio. All the activities of DNA, RNA, protein, and the whole system are always self-referral. When a mosquito comes and immediately the hand moves, it is the DNA that orders, "Look here! the danger is coming, you get up." This performance is self-referral because consciousness, intelligence, is developing itself into different expressions of its own nature and there is a continuity between matter and pure consciousness—the Self, the mind, and the body.

In this progression from Self to mind to body, we can look in finer detail at what happens at the transition point from subjectivity to objectivity. From the perspective of Panchamahabhuta theory in Maharishi Ayur-Ved, the finest level of matter in creation is described in terms of five basic constituents: *akash* (space), *vayu* (air), *agni* (fire), *jal* (water), and *prithivi* (earth). (The term *tejas* is also sometimes used for fire, the term *apas* for water. *Pancha* means "five"; thus the term *panchamahabhuta* means "five elements.") These five basic constituents have a subtle and a gross aspect. The subtle aspect is referred to as the five *tanmatras* and the gross aspect as the five *mahabhutas*. The five tanmatras are associated with the five senses. On the borderline between consciousness and matter, the senses are still within the subjective physiology of consciousness, and Maharishi explains that the tanmatras are the finest material expression of these five principles of nature:

The tanmatras constitute the five basic realities, or essences, of the objects of the five senses of perception. They express themselves in the five elements which go to make up the objects of the senses and which provide the material basis of the entire objective universe. Thus the essence of sound (*shabd* tanmatra) expresses itself in space, the essence of touch (*sparsh* tanmatra) in air, the essence of form (*rup* tanmatra) in fire, the essence of taste (*ras* tanmatra) in water, and the essence of smell (*gandh* tanmatra) in earth. . . . The tanmatras mark the dividing line between the subjective and objective creation. In the process of evolution, . . . the subjective creation comes to an end and the objective creation begins. The tanmatras, forming as they do the basis of the five elements, lie in the grossest field of the subjective aspect of creation.

The five mahabhutas (akash, vayu, etc.) are the same principles, found at a slightly more concrete level of the physiology of matter. Maharishi explains that they are the "elements out of which material creation is constituted"; the entire material creation evolves from these five fundamental elements. They are considered the building blocks from which matter arises.

In terms of our modern scientific understanding of the body, these concepts are perhaps more the concern of the most advanced and abstract areas of physics, having to do with the mechanics of nature that underlie biological functioning.

Dr. John Hagelin, director of the doctoral program in physics at Maharishi International University and one of the world's leading physicists in the area of unified quantum field theories, has interpreted the Panchamahabhuta theory in the terms of modern physics. Dr. Hagelin, who wrote the introduction to this book, is also an expert in Maharishi's Vedic Science and Technology, and in two recent articles, "Is Consciousness the Unified Field? A Field Theorist's Perspective," and "Restructuring Physics from its Foundation in Light of Maharishi's Vedic Science," he outlines the discovery of the unified field and its relationship to consciousness. In his discussion he makes use not only of the latest knowledge of modern quantum physics, but also of "the very complete description of the unified field and its self-interacting dynamics provided by Vedic Science as formulated by Maharishi Mahesh Yogi." In discussing the elementary particles and forces of nature, Dr. Hagelin explains that Maharishi's Vedic Science "provides a very natural and compact language of nature which is also based directly on the unified field."

In Dr. Hagelin's view, the transition from consciousness into matter in human life represents the junction point between the quantum mechanical and classical in the structure of the human physiology. He suggests that there is a distinct similarity between the five fundamental elements described in Maharishi's Vedic Science and Technology, and the fundamental spin types of quantum physics (he refers to the five elements as tanmatras rather than mahabhutas to emphasize their subtlest value). He first describes how, from the perspective of Maharishi's Vedic Science, the three-in-one dynamics of consciousness knowing itself (the Ved) generates "a rich spectrum of vibrational modes," which appear as all the forms and phenomena of the universe. Among these "resonant modes of consciousness," Dr. Hagelin points out, are the five fundamental categories of matter and energy—the tanmatras—responsible for the material universe. He further explains that

> there is a striking correspondence between these five tanmatras and the five quantum-mechanical spin types of a unified quantum field theory: between the akash or "space" tanmatra and the gravitational field; between the vayu or "air" tanmatra, which stands as a link between space and the other tanmatras, and the gravitino field; between the tejas or "fire" tanmatra, responsible for chemical transformations and the sense of sight, and the spin-1 force fields; and between the apas and prithivi ("water" and "earth") tanmatras and the spin-1/2 and spin-0 matter fields, respectively.

The figure on the following page presents Dr. Hagelin's brilliant insights into the structure the finest layers of creation, including the striking correspondences between the mechanics of natural law as described by the language of quantum field theory and in Maharishi's Vedic Science. The right side of the graphic depicts the emergence of the field of matter from the field of consciousness, as the three *doshas* (discussed in the next section) arise from the combinations of the five tanmatras.

Dr. Hagelin's recognition of the identity of the five elements described in Maharishi Ayur-Ved and in modern physics, as well as many other correspondences, is an important step in the growth of understanding of this knowledge in the scientific community. The process of connecting different fields of scientific knowledge to their

Structure of a Unified Quantum Field

GRAVITY SUPERFIELD *Vat*	GAUGE SUPERFIELDS *Pitt*	MATTER SUPERFIELDS *Kaph*

Spin-2 GRAVITON *Akash*

Spin-3/2 GRAVITINO *Vayu*

Spin-1 FORCES *Agni*

Spin-1/2 MATTER FIELDS *Jal*

Spin-0 HIGGS FIELDS *Prithivi*

Planck   **Scale**

Knower HILBERT SPACE *Rishi*

Process of Knowing OBSERVABLES *Devata*

Known STATES *Chhandas*

Intelligence QUANTUM PRINCIPLE

Existence FIELD

Unitary (string) dynamics *Samhita of the Ved*

This diagram presents Dr. John Hagelin's description of the fine mechanics of natural law by which the physical structure of creation emerges from the unified field of pure consciousness. It shows the correspondence between the fundamental aspects of intelligence described in Maharishi's Vedic Science and the structure of the laws of nature described in the language of quantum field theory. The right side of the diagram shows the three doshas arising from the five tanmatras. The blank boxes at the extreme right illustrate the elaboration of this sequential process of manifestation as it creates from these building blocks of matter the more manifest, concrete levels of physical creation.

source in the unified field of natural law is creating a bridge between modern science and Maharishi's Vedic Science that will allow scientists a more detailed and quantifiable understanding of how consciousness gives rise to matter.

The Three Doshas

According to Panchamahabhuta theory, the five elements combine to form three basic tendencies or operating principles of matter. These are known as the *doshas*. *Dosh** literally means "impurity." Doshas are considered impurities because as consciousness makes the transition from subjective to objective creation, it becomes "grosser" or more impure.

The three doshas are *vat,** *pitt*, and *kaph*. Vat, according to Ayurvedic texts, is a combination of akash and vayu; pitt, of agni and jal; and kaph, of jal and prithivi. In terms of the physiology, the three doshas represent three fundamental metabolic and psychophysiological principles underlying the functioning of the body, respectively: movement, metabolism, and structure.

The three doshas remind us of the three-in-one structure of pure consciousness, in which the three components—knower, process of knowing, and known—are called Rishi, Devata, and Chhandas. In fact, vat, pitt, and kaph are the finest material expressions in the body respectively of Rishi, Devata, and Chhandas.

According to Maharishi Ayur-Ved each person has a different proportion of the doshas at birth. In many respects, this is like saying that we each have a different mixture of genes. Although all three doshas are present in everyone, most people have primarily a combination of two of the three, with one predominating. (For example, one might be classified as a vat-pitt, vat-kaph, or pitt-kaph type.) Less common is the pure "mono-doshic" person, in which one dosh predominates. In rare instances, all three doshas may be equally in evidence.

Diet, age, weather, and countless other factors influence the proportion of doshas in the physiology. This has profound implications for health. When the doshas remain in their ideal proportion (which is dif-

---

* The "o" in *Dosh* is pronounced like the long "o" in doe. The "a" in *vat* is pronounced like the "a" in father.

ferent for different people), an individual remains healthy. When imbalance occurs—for example, if one of the doshas greatly increases or decreases in proportion to the others—the disease process begins. Susceptibility to different diseases, as well as the course of each disease, will vary depending upon which dosh predominates.

The goal of Maharishi Ayur-Ved is to recreate balance in vat, pitt, and kaph. When the doshas are balanced, the inner intelligence of the body is reflected more completely at all levels of physiological functioning.

How can we know the ideal proportion of doshas in the physiology? How can we diagnose their current state of balance? The traditional texts of Ayur-Ved describe three means of diagnosis: sight, speech, and touch. The first two involve a physical examination and interview to determine the patient's medical history and current symptoms. The subtlest diagnostic technique, however, is pulse diagnosis, traditionally called *nadi vigyan*. The *nadi*, or pulse, contains information about the patient's entire physical and mental condition.

Pulse Diagnosis in Maharishi Ayur-Ved

One of the greatest living experts in Maharishi Ayur-Ved is Dr. B. D. Triguna, past president of the All India Ayur-Veda Congress and member of the Indian government's Ayur-Veda research council. He is revered throughout his country and the world as a great *vaidya* (Ayurvedic physician), and a master of the subtle and sophisticated method of Ayurvedic pulse diagnosis. He was recently honored by the president of India with a special award for his long and distinguished career of devoted service to the health of the whole population.

On numerous occasions, I have been both surprised and impressed with Dr. Triguna's remarkable ability to diagnose disease through the pulse alone. Again and again he has diagnosed obscure conditions without any prior indication of the problem. On one occasion, a person was introduced and simply sat down. Dr. Triguna took his pulse and said, "This patient is colorblind." The man had indeed been colorblind since birth.

What does the physician detect in pulse diagnosis? It is certainly true that the pulse gives an overall indication of our heart and circulatory system. In Western medicine, one of the first diagnostic steps is to analyze the heart and circulatory system by measuring the pulse and taking the blood pressure. However, in Maharishi Ayur-Ved the diagnosis is far subtler and more comprehensive. When the physician puts his fingers on the radial pulse, he is not merely counting the number of pulses per minute as in Western medicine; he is determining the state of balance of the finer layers of the patient's physiology of matter.

The pulse in Maharishi Ayur-Ved is taken with three fingers: each finger is used to feel the state of one of the three doshas. The finger closest to the wrist determines the state of balance of vat, the middle finger determines the state of pitt, and the finger furthest from the wrist determines the state of kaph. The physician also feels the quality of the pulse—its strength, regularity, and rhythm—with all three fingers. By analyzing the state of balance of each dosh, the physician can determine many things about the patient and his state of health.

One thing the physician determines is the patient's Ayurvedic body type. We know that there are broad classifications of people—big, small, thin, muscular, fat, nervous, calm, etc.—yet modern medicine's knowledge of body or psychophysiological types is very rudimentary. If we go back to the historical roots of Western medicine, however, we do find a long tradition of body typing. Hippocrates, the father of Western medicine, and Galen, the great Roman physician, classified the temperament of patients according to the proportion of four basic bodily fluids—blood, yellow bile, black bile, and phlegm—the so-called four fundamental humors. Variations of this and other approaches were used from the Middle Ages to the nineteenth century by many famous physicians.

The first comprehensive and scientific approach to body typing in modern times was undertaken by W. H. Sheldon at Harvard University. In the 1930s and 1940s Dr. Sheldon surveyed a very large group of people and classified them into three main body types with many possible intermediate categories. These were named after the three main types of embryonic tissue from which all other tissues and organs eventually develop: the ectoderm, from which comes skin and nervous tissue; the mesoderm, from which muscle and connective tissue are derived; and the endoderm, from which most of our internal organs develop. Dr. Sheldon called the three basic types the ectomorph, the mesomorph, and endomorph. The ectomorph was in general tall and skinny, the mesomorph compact and muscular, and the endomorph fat and large. Dr. Sheldon also developed a very extensive scheme, involving many physical and psychological variables, for analyzing any individual according to the predominance or proportion of these three basic types. However, so far very little practical value has come from his research.

More recent attempts at classification are generally based on exclusively psychological characteristics. For example, the British psychologist Dr. Michael Eysenck developed the idea that people could be classified as introverts or extroverts. Perhaps the most successful modern psychosomatic typing is "Type A" coronary-prone behavior. As we discussed in Chapter 4, Type A's often display the negative behavioral characteristics of hostility, competitiveness, and hurriedness, and have been found in some studies to be more prone to heart disease.

Unfortunately none of these more recent attempts has taken advantage of the extensive knowledge and practical experience of Maharishi Ayur-Ved. The Ayurvedic system of health care contains extremely detailed knowledge of individual body types. Actually, they are more accurately called "mind-body" types, and by taking the pulse, the physician determines the natural psychophysiological makeup of an individual—the *prakriti*—which literally means "nature." An individual's prakriti represents the natural state of balance of the finer levels of the physiology of matter—the natural state of balance of the doshas (that is, the relative proportion of vat, pitt, and kaph).

Once the doctor knows the person's prakriti he can determine many factors. Most importantly he knows that each particular prakriti is susceptible to certain mental and physical disorders. The doctor can then, both from reading the pulse and also if necessary by physical examination, determine what is known as the *vikriti*. The vikriti is the deviation of the doshas from their ideal state of balance. Further, each dosh has five subdivisions, or subdoshas, within it. A physician skilled in Maharishi Ayur-Ved can determine which doshas and subdoshas are imbalanced and thereby give a precise analysis of the patient's particular disorder. Determining the vikriti is of great value even if no serious disorders are present, because the physician can detect in the subtle imbalances in the pulse the seeds of future health problems long before they manifest. Once the diagnosis is made, the Ayurvedic physician prescribes therapeutic and preventive strategies. Many of these are highly individualized, based on the patient's prakriti and vikriti.

From the viewpoint of Maharishi's Vedic Science, the ideal of Ayurvedic pulse diagnosis is when the vaidya feels the pulse, using the refined sense of touch, from the level of perfect balance and orderliness in his own highly developed awareness—from the level of his own self-interacting dynamics of consciousness. Starting from this level, his awareness precisely penetrates to the inner Self of the patient, fathoming the level where the infinite field of pure consciousness is becoming matter. From this level, he can thus feel the fluctuations of consciousness in the whole body.

A few years ago, Maharishi commented on Dr. Triguna's great skill in the art of pulse diagnosis, noting that it was a consequence of precisely this highly developed functioning of the great vaidya's awareness: "The miracle Dr. Triguna creates is that he just puts his fingers on that pulse where one is three. There, in the pulse, are those three values of observer, observed, and their relationship in the absolute unity of the three. This is how they diagnose which part of the system has become imbalanced. The heart, the brain, or whatever part is imbalanced is detected from the kind of pulse that a man has. Dr. Triguna has only to feel the pulse for two minutes and he can say, 'Your kidneys seem to be a little bit affected,' or, 'Your heart seems to be a little bit affected.' This sounds miraculous, but it is just the habit of measuring the quality of the pulse. It goes back to that transcendental, absolute level of the unified field where one is three."

From Maharishi's perspective it is the orderly awareness of the vaidya that enlivens orderliness within the disorder, or imbalance, present in the patient's doshas. In his view a great vaidya such as Dr. Triguna is functioning from this supreme level of diagnostic ability. This is clearly a completely new standard of medical performance to which any Western doctor would aspire. In fact, in the past few years many Western medical doctors have become trained in Maharishi Ayur-Ved and have been mastering the finer points of Ayuvedic pulse diagnosis as they apply it in their medical practices.

The Qualities of Vat, Pitt, and Kaph

To fully understand the body types in Maharishi Ayur-Ved we must understand the qualities of each of the three doshas: vat, pitt, and kaph.

The principle of vat, as we have said, arises from akash (space) and vayu (air). Vat is associated with movement within the body. It is involved with such vital functions as respiration, excretion, and neural control of sensory and motor function. People whose prakriti is predominantly vat (or "vat types") are characteristically thin and light. They are rarely comfortable in the cold, dislike strong wind, and prefer warm, balmy weather, warm water, and warm food. They have a marked tendency towards dry skin, some constipation, and a variable appetite, sometimes strong, sometimes weak.

Vat types tend to be bright, quick to grasp new concepts, quick to learn, but poor on long-term memory. Vatas are also quick to conceive and initiate projects, but have difficulty in following through to the end. They are often highly creative, but they can be overemotional, with extreme mood swings. When vatas feel good they can be almost euphoric.

When vat dosh goes out of balance, there is a strong tendency towards worry and anxiety. People prone to this imbalance often overextend themselves even though they lack profound physical strength and stability. Vat types are susceptible to arthritis and hypertension. In general, they have a high sensitivity to all environmental stimuli, with a low threshold of pain. A classic vat syndrome is well illustrated by the story of the princess and the pea. Even after 100 mattresses have been stacked on her bed, the princess is still disturbed by the presence of a tiny pea under the bottom mattress.

The second principal body type, pitt, is based on a predominance of pitt dosh in one's prakriti, which is associated with heat and metabolism. The elements of agni (fire) and jal (water) are the basis of pitt tendencies. Pitt is associated with such functions as digestion and thermoregulation. Pitt types share some of the characteristics of the vat types. They, too, tend to have agile minds; however, they have far more energy and staying power. They can be very aggressive, with a strong and penetrating intellect. They are well-organized and can be good, authoritative decision-makers. Their bodies can take a lot of physical discipline and abuse, and they frequently take overadvantage of this attribute. General George Patton was almost certainly a characteristic pitt type. It is not pure coincidence that military people and athletes are frequently found to be pitt types.

When pitt is imbalanced, pitt types will typically have trouble controlling their anger from time to time, if not frequently. They may be impatient and difficult to deal with. Pittas have strong digestion, but they must always have their food on time to maintain their equanimity. Peptic ulcer is the classic pitt health problem. Whenever a skin disorder appears, regardless of the individual's body type, it is an indication of a pitt imbalance. Pitt-type people have an aversion to hot weather and, regardless of weather, even the touch of their skin is noticeably warmer than that of a vat person.

The third principal body type, kaph, is based on a predominance of kaph dosh, which is associated with structure. In the fable of the tortoise and the hare, the tortoise is pure kaph—slow and steady wins the race. Within the body, kaph is concerned with the structural basis of the physiology. Its characteristics of solidity and inertia come from the elements of prithivi (earth) and jal (water). Structures such as membranes and connective tissue, which underlie the connectedness and stability of the body's different parts, are associated with kaph.

Kaph types tend to be more heavily built, with somewhat oily skin, and often have dark and thick hair. Digestion tends to be slow, and kaph people will often have a problem with overweight. Unlike vat types, they are not easily disturbed, and unlike pitt types, they are slow to anger. Their minds are tranquil and steady, slow to learn but slow to forget. Because they are not easily upset, they often are warm, forgiving, and agreeable. Negative tendencies of excess or imbalanced kaph can be dullness or sluggishness and the lack of creativity and ambition. Kaphas enjoy their heavy and deep sleep, but must have enough to be lively and focused the next day. The most predominant kaph health disorders are asthma and obesity.

Considering the potential importance of psychophysiological or body typing, it is remarkable that so little scientific research has been conducted in this area. Perhaps this is because of the great variability among individuals, or the lack of a fundamental understanding of the very real physiological foundation of such a diagnostic framework. As we have mentioned, research has been conducted on Type A and Type B coronary-prone behavior, but researchers are justifiably cautious about its accuracy and therefore its effectiveness as a reliable diagnostic tool.

I believe that the understanding provided by Maharishi Ayur-Ved could give the proper theoretical basis for a thorough scientific investigation of this area. Preliminary laboratory evidence is very revealing. In one study, subjects were assessed according to the procedures of Maharishi Ayur-Ved and also for Type A and B behavior. Significant correlations were found between individuals with a predominantly pitt (and to a lesser extent vat) constitution and the Type A coronary-prone behavior pattern, and between those with kaph constitution and the Type B behavior pattern, which is less prone to heart disease. In addition, kaph-type people had significantly higher cholesterol and triglyceride levels than vat people. Further, significant differences were also found in measurements of pulse rate, white blood cell counts, and EEG frequencies.

One of the most interesting investigations concerning the physiological basis of Ayurvedic body types was conducted in India by researchers at the University of Benares. In these studies an attempt was made to correlate the three main Ayurvedic body types with blood levels of three principal neurotransmitters. The findings over several studies indicate that the vat type has significantly higher levels of acetylcholine; the pitt, higher levels of norepinephrine; and the kaph, higher levels of histamine.

Further research should provide a fuller physiological understanding of the Ayurvedic psychophysiological typing system and thus help to introduce it more widely to the West. On the basis of this system, Maharishi Ayur-Ved provides a comprehensive nutritional and dietary program specifically designed for each type. Further, it gives specific advice and procedures in regard to behavior, lifestyle, and physical fitness. Extensive knowledge exists in Maharishi Ayur-Ved concerning daily and seasonal biological rhythms with regard to individual body type. On this basis certain daily and seasonal routines are prescribed for better health.

Let's consider why the knowledge of someone's body type is valuable. Take the example of Anne, who was diagnosed as being angry. The modern physician, if he made the correct diagnosis, wouldn't really have much to offer such a patient. He probably would prescribe some mild sedative, or, if the condition worsened, a tranquillizer or painkiller. He might refer the patient to a psychologist or psychiatrist, who would probably prescribe more sophisticated medication.

Maharishi Ayur-Ved, on the other hand, would treat the patient very differently. In Maharishi Ayur-Ved, as in most systems of natural medicine, the orientation is toward the patient, not the disease. Who is my patient? What is his or her body type? What are the tendencies towards imbalances that cause physical or mental disorders? After examining the patient, taking the pulse, and fully evaluating the patient's body type, the physician would probably find, as in the case of Anne, that she was a pitt type. This would explain her tendency towards anger.

Further, the physician would question what foods the person had been eating. Certain foods are known to increase pitt and can actually cause anger to be expressed more quickly. He would also examine other relevant aspects of the patient's life that might also aggravate pitt and further note the time of day and season, since both these factors affect how the pitt-type person is behaving. Western-trained physicians who are also trained in Maharishi Ayur-Ved are inevitably impressed by the importance of understanding the patient's body type before trying to prescribe a treatment or prevention program.

Balance

Each body type has its own strengths and weaknesses, and each person has his own genetic makeup and his own relative proportion of vat, pitt, and kaph. Whatever that proportion is, it should be maintained in balance. According to Maharishi Ayur-Ved, disease occurs only when these three fundamental psychophysiological principles— vat, pitt, and kaph—become aggravated or imbalanced.

Maharishi Ayur-Ved describes the various stages of imbalance that lead to disease. Perhaps most interesting, what we would consider in Western medicine to be a disorder's early symptoms are, in fact, the last stages in Maharishi Ayur-Ved. Through the knowledge of body types and the three doshas, physicians are able to detect much earlier stages of disease.

For example, they may detect an imbalance caused by an excess of pitt building up in some area of the body. There may be general symptoms of irritability or anger, but it is impossible at this stage to know how the disease will actually manifest. If the buildup becomes too great, then, according to Maharishi Ayur-Ved, some area of the body that is weaker and more prone to a pitt imbalance will become the target for the excess pitt. Instead of remaining a nonlocal mild state of weakness, the disturbance suddenly becomes localized and perhaps inflamed, causing the target organ or tissue to develop acute symptoms of a particular disease.

Since one site prone to pitt imbalance is the stomach area, the patient might develop indigestion or even ulcers. These are just a few of the common signs of pitt imbalance; it is important to note that symptoms can arise from imbalances in any of the doshas. The physician trained in Maharishi Ayur-Ved takes many different factors into account when diagnosing disorders and prescribing treatment for them.

In terms of modern medicine, we might understand this process of balance and imbalance in terms of one of the most important physiological principles—the principle of homeostasis. Homeostasis refers to the body's ability to maintain internal balance and stability even when there are changes in the environment.

There are many such mechanisms to keep all parts of our body in balance. Thus, the importance of balance is well understood in modern medicine. If one of these regulatory mechanisms is disturbed or overtaxed, for example in states of physical and mental stress, then the whole system suffers. Maharishi Ayur-Ved has very refined procedures for detecting these physiological imbalances and treating them before they actually manifest into a particular disease; this is one aspect of its successful prevention-oriented approach to health care.

Individual Dietary Needs: Food is Medicine

In Maharishi Ayur-Ved, food is regarded as medicine. It would be unheard of to prescribe a treatment for a particular disorder without taking into consideration first, the individual's body type, and second, the particular foods that would be beneficial in correcting the physiological imbalance and preventing new ones from arising.

This is in great contrast to our current tradition of nutrition, which emphasizes an ideal or "best" diet for everyone. Of course, this best diet is constantly changing. Every few months, new best-selling diet books are prominently displayed across the country. Does anyone ever wonder why more and more books keep appearing? It must be for one of two reasons. Either there is a steady stream of brilliant Nobel prize–level scientific research being done in this area, or none of these new diet plans really works, so people keep trying new and "better" ones.

Most of the modern medical profession would agree with the latter. Quick and easy diet plans can sometimes produce some initial results, but in the long run the best approach seems to be a slow and steady process tailored to each individual and based on factors such as lifestyle and exercise.

If everyone is not already confused enough about new diet plans, what about the health food vitamin books? This is an area of huge controversy, not only between the medical profession and health food experts, but even among all the different health food experts themselves. Diet and nutrition probably have more self-styled "experts" than any other health-related area. Who can you believe? Will vitamin C cure my cold? Will selenium protect us against cancer? These are some of the many issues that no one seems able to agree upon.

The health food people say the medical profession is too conservative and wants to control everything; therefore, it doesn't let the public in on the latest scientific findings. The medical profession is equally critical of the health food people, saying that based on only a few animal studies—or even without any research whatsoever—extraordinary and unsubstantiated claims are made for various vitamins, minerals, etc. The problem is that in both cases the conclusions about diet are based on incomplete knowledge, or knowledge that is constantly changing.

For example, in recent years the American Heart Association has been urging every person to reduce or give up saturated fats in milk, cheese, butter, and meat in favor of polyunsaturated fats. "Polyunsaturated" has become the byword for selling margarine and cooking oil for years. However, more recent research suggests that excess polyunsaturated fats may cause an increase in free radical reactions. This is a type of chemical reaction that may be at the basis of many disorders, including cancer and aging (free radicals are discussed further in Chapters 7 and 8). More and more doctors are now recommending that a balance of fats be included in the diet, with monosaturated fats at the top of the list and polyunsaturated fats at the bottom. Yet many Americans still routinely buy polyunsaturated oils thinking that they are protecting their health.

Maharishi Ayur-Ved:
A Time-Tested Tradition of Nutrition

Maharishi Ayur-Ved places great emphasis on diet. Many foods and spices are considered to have important value for health, and therefore are recommended along with other treatment modalities. The most important difference between Maharishi Ayur-Ved and modern nutrition is Maharishi Ayur-Ved's concern for individual differences. If we were to analyze the various Maharishi Ayur-Ved diets, we would find that virtually all them conform to what modern nutritionists consider a balanced diet. They contain the right proportion and quality of fats, protein, minerals, vitamins, and carbohydrates. However, Maharishi Ayur-Ved very clearly states that no one diet is right for all people. What is considered nourishing for one individual can actually be detrimental to another.

For example, some sweets are said to be good for the vat type, while for a kaph type they may cause respiratory congestion or excess fat. Hot, spicy foods are very good for kaphas, yet they aggravate the digestion of a pitt type, leading to indigestion and a marked tendency towards anger. Each individual type has its own needs.

Spontaneously, most of us have noticed over the years that certain types of food seem to be bad for us or are less appealing. On the other hand, sometimes we eat them anyway even though we know they have bad effects on us. This could be because of imbalance, habit, ignorance, or failure to listen to the messages our physiology gives us. Maharishi Ayur-Ved provides a reliable, systematic body of knowledge that explains why we should or should not have certain types of food. Maharishi Ayur-Ved is based on a long tradition of practical experience and a profound theoretical basis. But because of our often superior attitude toward "folk medicines," the dietary principles of traditional medical systems have unfortunately never been scientifically studied.

According to Maharishi Ayur-Ved, an important consideration when determining our diet is the strength of our digestion. Each body type has a different strength of digestion, which is also influenced by factors such as climate and one's age and state of health. Most importantly, digestive strength depends upon the activity of our *agnis*. The agnis are the "fires of digestion," perhaps equivalent to our modern understanding of digestive enzymes. Weak agnis and improperly digested food can be a source of imbalance in the doshas. The by-product of undigested food is a substance which Ayur-Ved calls *ama*. The accumulation of ama aggravates the doshas and leads to all types of disorders.

The concept of disease caused by undigested food products is similar to many early theories on the aging process, which suggested that aging was caused by the accumulation of toxic materials in the colon. A more recent study on aging suggested that the waste products from bacteria in the colon, known as endotoxins, can modify certain activities of the immune system. This suppression of the immune system would correspond to the imbalance of the doshas as described in Maharishi Ayur-Ved. More research in this important area of digestion should help us understand some of the traditional Ayurvedic concepts in the framework of modern terminology.

Body Type and Exercise

One of the most visible signs of the growing trend towards self-improvement in health is the fitness craze. Particularly in the United States during the past decade or so, more and more people have been taking up jogging, aerobics, or body building, or are involved in some type of diet or physical fitness program. There is a steady stream not only of diet, but also of exercise and fitness books. One can't help but see this as a healthy sign. People are at least waking up and remembering what it's like to get outside, breathe fresh air, and get the body moving again. The only trouble is that like many other things we do in America, we overdo. What started out as a positive direction of improving health has turned in many cases into a compulsive and over-taxing burden on our bodies.

It's remarkable how much damage can be caused to the body from something as simple as jogging. Studies have made it clear that all kinds of bone, joint, and back problems can result from excessive, incorrect, or compulsive jogging programs. Other fitness programs as well can produce bad side effects, primarily because of our over-enthusiastic desire to immediately become fit, or because we are not physically prepared or capable of doing them.

Maharishi Ayur-Ved again emphasizes the need to structure any exercise program according to age and body type. Up to the age of 25, moderate to vigorous exercise on a regular basis is prescribed for all body types. Over the age of 25, Ayur-Ved generally advises more moderate exercise for all types, with the following specific recommendations for each type.

Kaph types are the best suited for vigorous exercise, and it is essential that they exercise regularly. Otherwise, they will gain weight and tend to become lethargic. Pitt types are often strong, muscular, and well-suited for exercise. For them moderate exercise is prescribed on a regular basis. Pitt people, like Type A individuals, have a tendency to overdo it. When exercising, they should not allow their competitive and sometimes driven spirit to push their physiologies too far, well beyond their normal capacities. This holds especially true for team sports. The vat type is more suited for very moderate exercise maintained on a regular basis. The vat type, in particular, needs to be careful about engaging in a fitness program that might be too strenuous. For vat types some of these programs could be detrimental, causing exhaustion, rather than beneficial.

Walking is one exercise recommended for all body types. Other specific exercises are also recommended for all body types. The most well-known of these are the *Yog asanas*, a series of easy postures that stimulate the body in a systematic and natural way. Specific asanas can be recommended by Maharishi Ayur-Ved physicians to enhance the treatment of particular disorders.

The goal of all exercise in Maharishi Ayur-Ved is to rejuvenate the body and create bliss. Exercise should not be a strain to the physiology. The saying "no pain, no gain" is replaced by "gain without pain." For athletes, Maharishi Ayur-Ved prescribes effective training programs for optimizing performance without causing the physical discomfort and negative side effects characteristic of so many other programs. Dr. John Douillard, who is Associate Director of the Maharishi Ayur-Ved Health Center in Lancaster, Massachusetts, also directs its Ayurvedic sports and fitness programs. He explains the main principle behind these programs:

> The body has full, unlimited potential. It is the stress and fatigue of exertion that inhibit the athlete from reaching full athletic potential. When you remove the strain and fatigue, you remove the inhibiting factors. Once the stress and impurities are gone, then the athlete can perform at peak level. In fact, with Ayurvedic exercise, the potential for performance is unlimited.

The Maharishi Ayur-Ved approach to athletic training, which is employed in the Invincible Athletics Course, leads to much higher performance levels. Dr. Douillard, a former professional triathlete who competed in "ironman" marathons, has taught these Ayurvedic techniques to a number of well-known professional athletes. For both the average exercise buff and the professional athlete alike, Maharishi Ayur-Ved considers all aspects of the individual to create "a sound mind in a sound body."

Biological Rhythms

A vital part of almost all traditional systems of medicine is a knowledge of biological rhythms. Maharishi Ayur-Ved draws on a long-standing tradition that includes an especially rich and extensive knowledge of the impact of biological rhythms on diet, treatment of disease, behavior, and numerous other factors related to the individual body type. In modern medicine we have only recently verified the importance of biological rhythms and, as a result, the field of chronobiology—the study of biological rhythms—has received widespread attention.

The most obvious biological rhythm is the diurnal or circadian rhythm, which results from the rotation of the earth about its axis every 24 hours. Many of our vital physiological signs, such as internal body temperature, as well as many biochemical and hormone levels, follow a daily pattern. Within our brain is an internal clock that helps keep track of time and set rhythms. Scientists have found a number of chronobiotic agents that can affect our daily rhythms. The most obvious of these are the environmental patterns of periods of light and dark that constantly reset our internal clock to match our environment. Also important are the foods we eat, the drugs and stimulants (such as coffee) we take, and the times we eat, rest, and exercise.

Anyone who has ever travelled knows that the biological resetting process, commonly referred to as "jet lag," can be very tiring and taxing. In the same way, we are all too aware of what happens if we stay up too late one night or miss meals. We put a strain on the body's own natural rhythms and, as a result, we create a temporary imbalance in the physiology, which must be corrected later on. Health, memory, emotions, job performance, and motor coordination have all been shown to be affected by shifts in our daily rhythms.

Perhaps the most important findings have been those related to modern medical treatment. Studies have shown that some drugs work differently at different times of the day. Dr. Franz Halberg, a pioneer in chronobiology, was one of the first scientists to document the importance of timing when treating cancer with radiation or with drugs.

Dr. Halberg found that a dose of radiation that killed mice at one time of day was much less toxic at another time. The tumor cells themselves were more sensitive to radiation at different times of the day. In the late 1960s he and his colleagues showed dramatic improvements in treating mouth tumors by properly timing the radiation treatment. Since these early studies, numerous other studies have shown that the timing of both radiation and chemotherapy can make a marked difference in the effectiveness of the treatment. Drugs work at so many different levels of the physiology of matter, and each level has its own biological rhythm. DNA synthesis has its own rhythm, as do all the hormones, biochemicals, and even the cardiovascular system. For example, heart attacks strike three times more often at 9 A.M. than at 11 P.M.

The importance of understanding the body's biorhythms applies not only to the treatment of disease but also to its diagnosis. For example, there are numerous fluctuations in blood pressure as a result of its biological rhythms. Yet in a doctor's office, usually only one measurement at one time of the day is made to determine whether a patient has high blood pressure. It is easy to understand why misdiagnosis may occur. Some researchers have measured fluctuations in blood pressure and have used this information in diagnosis. For example, researchers have found that the pattern of these fluctuations in newborns can be used to predict their chances of developing high blood pressure when they grow older.

Maharishi Ayur-Ved takes into account varying biological rhythms in all phases of diagnosis, prevention, and treatment. It also takes into account the interaction of body type and diet with these rhythms. The principal goal of Maharishi Ayur-Ved is to establish balance. Thus it places a special significance on establishing harmony between our individual rhythms and those of nature through various daily and seasonal routines. When we get out of the city into the countryside, we immediately notice the impact of nature's regularity. All the birds and animals wake up at a regular time; nature functions in a systematic and routine way. It should come as no surprise, then, that we are also designed to follow nature's rhythms. Maharishi Ayur-Ved therefore utilizes various therapeutic programs (which we will describe in the next chapter) that reset our biological clocks to be in tune with those of nature.

The Effects of Seasonal Cycles on Our Health

One consideration in Maharishi Ayur-Ved quite new to Western understanding is the interaction of season, diet, and disease. While our current scientific understanding of seasonal changes is far from complete, recent research, especially on the pineal gland (as we mentioned in Chapter 3), has shown that animals are very sensitive to seasonal changes. As the day becomes longer, the amount of light stimulation increases. This has an effect on the secretion of melatonin, which in turn regulates other key glands, especially those involved in reproduction. Modern medicine has uncovered some of the ways these seasonal changes might influence our health. For example, a condition known as seasonal affective disorder (SAD), which results in depression, occurs especially in northern countries and is caused by lack of sunlight, which influences the activity of the pineal gland.

According to Maharishi Ayur-Ved, seasonal changes can increase susceptibility to a number of disorders. The type of disorder can depend on the season and our body type. The seasons themselves are related to the different doshas. This is because in Maharishi's Vedic Science, the same laws of nature—the expressions of Rishi, Devata, and Chhandas—are found not only in the human physiology but also at every level of the environment. Thus even the seasons reflect the governing principles of vat, pitt, and kaph.

For example, at the beginning of kaph season (early spring), the weather is often cold and damp and therefore more likely to cause an increase in kaph. Especially in kaph-type people, this can create an imbalance resulting in colds, bronchitis, etc. On the other hand, at the beginning of pitt season (early summer) pitt types, who are generally "hot" to begin with, may become imbalanced, leading to increased digestive problems and bouts of anger. Vat types are most susceptible to disease in vat season, the cold and windy winter months. To protect the individual during these times of greater susceptibility, Maharishi Ayur-Ved makes many dietary and behavioral recommendations for each body type.

The Vedic seers knew that the rhythms of the human body were tied to the rhythms of nature. They knew that for each person there was an ideal daily and seasonal routine to ensure that his or her rhythms were continually reset and resynchronized with those of the earth, moon, and sun. Further, they knew that the timing of a medical treatment was critical to its success. Therefore, all Maharishi Ayur-Ved treatments are individualized not only for the body type, but for the time of day, the season, and the age of the patient.

Maharishi's Vedic Science emphasizes that ideal health can only exist on the basis of an ideal relationship between human life and the laws of nature. The knowledge of the fundamental structures of the physiology of matter and of the physiology of consciousness—and of their underlying unity within the state of pure consciousness—provides a clear framework with which we can understand the technologies of the Vedic paradigm. This knowledge points to the reality that we, at a most fundamental level, are intimately connected with nature. It shows us that in the very process of realigning ourselves with the laws of nature, we can transform our personal experience and the world around us; we can transform our very physiologies. Maharishi uses a simple analogy to describe this relationship:

> It should be firmly established in the mind of every individual that he is part of the whole life of the universe and that his relationship to universal life is that of one cell to the whole body . . . . The boundaries of the individual life are not restricted to the boundaries of the body, nor even to those of one's family or one's home. They extend far beyond those spheres to the limitless horizon of unbounded cosmic life.

CHAPTER 6

THE NETWORK OF INTELLIGENCE

A FEW YEARS AGO I WAS INVITED TO SPEAK AT A PHYSICIANS' conference at the Maharishi Ayur-Ved Health Center in Lancaster, Massachusetts. As I drove up the long driveway to the health center, surrounded by many acres of snowy woods, I felt pleased to be in New England once again. Although I was born in California, my real roots are in New England, where I spent years as a youth and where most of my relatives still live.

New England is also one source of my deep interest in health and human physiology. My grandfather, who had a strong influence on all my family, was a pioneer in his field, a surgeon who graduated from Harvard Medical School, worked with the Mayo brothers, and was a founding member of the New England Surgical Society. After performing several historic operations he established his own hospital in Fall River, Massachusetts. To me he represents the good that modern medicine stands for.

So it was natural for me in this New England setting to think of how my grandfather might have regarded the Vedic paradigm and its applications to health. I am sure that he, like most physicians, would have thought it strange at first that modern medicine was forced to go back in time and restore an ancient tradition of knowledge in order to become more complete and effective. However, I think that if he could have been there at the conference and heard about the numerous research studies and the full range of medical strategies available, he would have been keenly interested.

Dr. Tony Nader, co-director of the Lancaster center, was participating in the conference to present the first research on Maharishi Ayur Ved—the first verification by Western science of the benefits of this most ancient system of natural health care. These findings, which will be discussed in detail in the next chapter, showed the extraordinary practical value of several herbal preparations of Maharishi Ayur-Ved. Most striking about Dr. Nader's findings was the potentially wide application of these herbal preparations for promoting health and longevity.

Maharishi Ayur-Ved is a complete approach to health care which emphasizes prevention rather than cure, the patient rather than the disease. The physician focuses not only on the symptoms of illness in a patient, but on creating a complete state of balance in the mind, physiology, and behavior. Maharishi Ayur-Ved emphasizes the proper interaction of—and the balance between—mind and body, consciousness and matter. The many therapeutic strategies of Maharishi Ayur-Ved, including herbal preparations, are oriented toward strengthening the patient's own natural defenses against disease. These strategies are designed to unfold and express the inner intelligence of the body—to reconnect the body with its basis in consciousness and thus help the body heal itself.

Maharishi Ayur-Ved has restored the importance of consciousness and its inner dynamics to our understanding of human physiology and health. It has reconnected the individual with nature, locating in our own mind and body the source of natural law in the universe. It has also provided us with the very practical and scientifically validated technologies of twenty-five approaches with which we can improve health and increase longevity.

Before we discuss some of these approaches, it is important to understand a key concept in the Vedic paradigm—the mistake of the intellect.

The Mistake of the Intellect

In Chapter 5, we discussed the principle of balance and imbalance in Maharishi Ayur-Ved. Now let's go a little deeper into this concept and see its basis in the fine mechanics of natural law.

In the Vedic paradigm, it is the intellect that inhibits us most from seeing our true inner nature, and it is the intellect that is ultimately responsible for our state of health.

The intellect has the ability to shift our attention in one of two directions: either outward toward the diversity of life, or inward toward the unity of consciousness. Maharishi's Vedic Science refers to a condition known as *pragyaparadh*, the "mistake of the intellect." In this condition, the intellect becomes so absorbed in the diversified value of creation that it cannot perceive the underlying unity of life. According to Maharishi Ayur-Ved, this is the basic cause of imbalance in the physiology. To eliminate this mistake, we must reawaken within our awareness its underlying unified value. We must shift our attention to the wholeness of consciousness by using strategies that are able to realign every aspect of the physiology of matter with the most fundamental level of our physiology of consciousness.

Another way to understand this is that illness and physiological imbalances are due to distortions in the sequential unfoldment of natural law. At the level of pure consciousness, natural law is constantly and spontaneously unfolding itself through the self-interacting dynamics of consciousness.

We remember from our earlier discussion that pure consciousness, in the act of knowing itself, creates within itself the three-in-one structure of Samhita (unified value) of Rishi (knower), Devata (process of knowing), and Chhandas (known). The mutual interactions of Samhita, Rishi, Devata, and Chhandas produce a series of sequential transformations, through which emerges the Ved—all the laws of nature that structure and govern the whole universe.

Addressing an international conference on Maharishi Ayur-Ved in Washington, D.C., several years ago, Maharishi explained that the self-referral nature of pure consciousness, the unified field of natural law, is what gives it the quality of perfect balance: "The unified field is perfectly balanced because its status is self-referral, its activity self-interacting. . . . It cannot be disturbed. It is a state of eternal balance, which is the ideal of balance. . . . "

As natural law sequentially expresses itself, it creates the structures of the physiology of consciousness, and finally of the physiology of matter. As we have seen, the doshas and all the body's material structures are the concrete expressions of Rishi, Devata, and Chhandas. At the conference, Maharishi went on to explain that, because the unified field is the basis of all the structures of the body, they also reflect its state of perfect balance:

> The Self, intellect, mind, senses, body, and all the different organs of the body—all that is self-referral. From DNA to RNA to proteins to the different systems of the body—the entire performance is completely self-referral. . . . As that unified state expresses itself into diversity, the intellect aspect—which is one with the Self—spontaneously and most naturally modifies itself and is expressed in different modes or qualities of life. In our own structure, we have eyes that only see, ears that only hear, touch that only touches—different qualities or characteristics in our body, and all are completely balanced. The functioning of the eyes and ears and speech is balanced just because of the basic self-referral character of life in the unified field, the self-referral state of intelligence.

Maharishi further explained that imbalances arise in the body, leading to pain, sickness, and suffering, whenever the process of manifestation of intelligence into matter loses its self-referral quality—that is, becomes disconnected from the underlying unity of life:

> Balance is the natural state of life. Life is always balanced because the basic characteristic of its fundamental element, the unified field, is complete balance. In the process of expansion of the unified field, consciousness becomes matter and matter assumes different characteristics. If in this process imbalances come along, then the coordination between mind and some aspect of the body breaks.
>
> This breaking of coordination is also a natural process. We have seen how the three-fold structure of the Ved—Rishi, Devata, and Chhandas—breaks from their unity. This is the fundamental feat of spontaneous dynamical symmetry breaking, as it is called in quantum field theory. Because this breaking of symmetry is a natural phenomenon, imbalance is also a natural phenomenon. Balance is a natural phenomenon and gaining the state of imbalance is also a natural phenomenon. Balance is a state of satisfaction. Deviation from balance is dissatisfaction. Pain and suffering result from imbalances. Anywhere in the process of manifestation of intelligence into matter or in the reaction of matter with matter, anywhere in those space-time boundaries that the self-referral condition is unavailable, there is pain and suffering.

The intellect, Maharishi pointed out, plays the central role in maintaining balance, by maintaining its complete coordination with the Self. "If some abnormality develops in the intellect, then, even if something is right, one would comprehend it to be wrong. It is the fineness of the intellect which maintains the self-referral state. In this state the intellect is completely coordinated with the Self. There the three values of Rishi, Devata, and Chhandas . . . emerge from one state of Samhita. If the intellect is in a balanced state then everything is brilliant, clear, full of satisfaction, and blissful."

The diagram on the following page shows how pragyaparadh arises in the context of this understanding of the sequential unfoldment of natural law. Through the mistake of the intellect, the diverse expressions of the self-referral intelligence in our physiology of consciousness "forget" their basis in the unmanifest, unified state of pure consciousness. The Samhita, or unity value of pure consciousness, is lost to our view; the doshas—the expressions of Rishi, Devata, and Chhandas in the body—lose their connection to their source, and thus they become imbalanced. When imbalances arise in the physiology of consciousness, they in turn create (for example, through improper diet and poor daily routine) imbalances and disease in the physiology of matter.

The purpose of the twenty approaches of Maharishi Ayur-Ved is to reset the sequential unfoldment of the expressions of natural law in our physiology of matter. They fulfill this purpose by helping us attune ourselves to the most fundamental level of our physiology of consciousness—pure consciousness, the state of perfect balance. This process of resetting automatically corrects the mistake of the intellect, since it enables us to wake up to our own inner Self.

This is how we can spontaneously and automatically restore perfect balance in the physiology. The inner intelligence of the body, the "memory" of the unified value of pure consciousness, is reawakened, and the body's own homeostatic mechanisms begin to function optimally, thus eliminating disease, restoring health, and promoting longevity.

Maharishi explains how the purpose of Maharishi Ayur-Ved to promote longevity is fulfilled by maintaining "that state of Samhita, that state of togetherness of the fundamental values of life":

> That is the state of immortality. Rishi, Devata, and Chhandas in their coordinated value maintain Samhita, the Ved, in an immortal state.

Ved is immortal. Pure knowledge is immortal. The organizing power of nature inherent in the structure of pure knowledge is immortal. Thus balance is immortal, and if, through the knowledge of Ayur-Ved, one maintains balance in the physiology, mind, and behavior, then that is the direction of long life.

Primordial Sound

In the study of human development, we know that exact, sequential, and predictable physical and mental changes occur as a human being evolves from a fertilized egg to birth, adolescence, adulthood, and old age. While there are variations on the theme of human development, there is an underlying score. And the entire process is orchestrated by DNA.

In terms of the Vedic paradigm, the "sequential unfoldment" of DNA takes on a deeper meaning. All processes in the physiology—and indeed all processes in the universe—have a common basis in pure consciousness, the unified field of all the laws of nature. The laws of nature, the patterns of intelligence and creativity inherent in pure consciousness, manifest as subjectivity and objectivity—as the physiology of consciousness and the physiology of matter—in an orderly and predictable way.

We have seen how natural law unfolds through a series of transformations in pure consciousness which, Maharishi explains, express dif-

Pragyaparadh: The Source of All Disorder and Disease

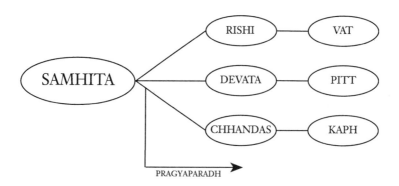

98

ferent frequencies of self-interaction. What is the nature of these different frequencies? Maharishi explains that they are actually frequencies of *sound*—the "hum" of the vibration produced by the self-interacting dynamics of pure consciousness as it transforms itself from one mode into another.

Another name for these unmanifest sounds within pure consciousness is *primordial sounds*. In Maharishi's explanation, primordial sounds are "the language of nature,"—the sounds created by the unified field interacting within itself. The Ved is the name given to the precise, perfectly orderly sequence of primordial sounds that expresses the complete unfoldment of natural law from pure consciousness. As Maharishi states, "The Ved in its original script is just the whisper of the unified field to itself."

Now we have a fuller context in which to understand our explanation in Chapter 1, that Vedic literature is the "script" of this sequential unfoldment of the laws of nature. As Maharishi explains, "Ved is a clear script of that self-interacting situation of pure consciousness. Nature in its absolutely pure state is very clear in its precise activity, its precise performance, and that is the Ved." The Vedic literature is the record of the primordial sounds of nature, the patterns of intelligence unfolding within pure consciousness and eventually creating the structures of matter and the body.

According to Maharishi Ayur-Ved, it is primordial sounds that structure and direct all matter and energy. They are the basic impulses of natural law that are responsible for all creation. Like seeds about to sprout, these impulses of nature's intelligence are not yet manifest, but are vibrating within themselves, forming the dynamic, self-referral fabric of the unified field. This unmanifest fabric of primordial sound is the basis of our own physiology of consciousness.

Contained in seed form in primordial sounds is the blueprint of the manifest universe, in the same way that DNA contains in seed form the blueprint of the entire body. There is an intimate relationship between the unmanifest seed sounds in consciousness and their manifest expressions in matter. The Vedic paradigm calls this the relationship of *nam* (name) and *rup* (form): the name is composed of different sounds—different frequencies of self-interaction; the form is the material expression that spontaneously arises from the sequential unfoldment of the sound or name. In other words, the form is simply a more manifest expression of the vibratory impulses in the name.

Again, we can see an analogous situation in DNA, where each gene within the DNA codes for a specific protein. The name is the information coded in the sequence of nucleotides on the DNA, and the form is the three-dimensional shape of the particular protein.

Primordial sounds are the basis of one of the twenty-five approaches of Maharishi Ayur-Ved, which makes use of this intimate relationship between the seed sounds and their manifest forms in the body. The body, at its finest level, is just the expression of primordial sound. As we just saw, disease and disorders arise due to pragyaparadh, when the material forms in the body become disconnected from their self-referral basis in pure consciousness. That is, the sequential unfoldment of primordial sounds has been disrupted, has gotten out of its proper sequence.

The primordial sound approach of Maharishi Ayur-Ved is designed to reset the unfoldment of intelligence in our body to match its original perfect pattern in pure consciousness, and thus to remove any physiological imbalances. This principle of resetting the correct unfoldment of intelligence lies at the heart of the therapeutic strategies of Maharishi Ayur-Ved.

By way of analogy, consider an orchestra rehearsing Beethoven's Symphony no. 7. There is a perfect orderliness and beauty in the musical piece, which is represented on a gross manifest level by the notes on the musical score. The conductor, the "DNA" of the orchestra, has in his awareness exactly how the piece should unfold and how all the instruments should relate to each other; he is responsible for the orderly unfoldment of the intelligence in the music. At any stage of the piece, he can identify if a note is played out of sequence, or if a wrong note has been played. The conductor compares what is being played to the pattern of the unmanifest musical score that he holds in his awareness. If an error occurs, he stops the rehearsal and indicates where a correction must be made. In this activity, he is actually reconnecting the performance of the orchestra with the patterns of musical intelligence in his own awareness. He enlivens this intelligence in the awareness of the musicians; they spontaneously correct their performance, and the music proceeds. This process resets the perfect sequential unfoldment of the music.

In the physiology, we can see how this principle operates in the development of cancer: cancer cells are renegade cells that have declared mutiny on the body. The sequence of expression of knowledge in DNA (the name) has become distorted; as a result their material form also becomes distorted, as well as dangerous. The cells have lost their memory of what they are supposed to do, and instead of functioning as normal cells, they produce large quantities of growth factors and begin to divide and spread at an unchecked rate, exhausting the body's resources for their growth.

The use of primordial sound is designed to reconnect the material structure of the physiology with the self-referral intelligence at its basis. This enlivenment of the inner intelligence of the body helps the body to spontaneously heal itself. In the case of cancer, the sequence of the expression of DNA would regain its normal pattern, and the cells would thus regain their memory of how to function as healthy cells.

Researchers at Ohio State University have found experimental evidence suggesting that the primordial sounds of the Vedic literature have a beneficial effect on re-enlivening the inner intelligence of the body. The effects of primordial sound were compared to those of hard rock music, and no sound, on the growth of cells in culture. Five types of human cancer cells (lung, colon, brain, breast, and melanoma) and one normal cell type were tested in four experiments. The recordings of primordial sound and hard rock were adjusted so that the degree of loudness was similar for both. Primordial sound decreased growth in all the cancer cell types. In the presence of hard rock music, cell growth was generally increased, although the effects were not consistent.

In Maharishi Ayur-Ved there is also a mental technique called Primordial Sound therapy, which prescribes specific primordial sounds according to the specific physiological disorder. As the impulses of primordial sound reverberate in the awareness, a kind of sympathetic resonance occurs; they act as a template that can restore the body to a state of balance.

Discovery of the Ved in Human Physiology

Before I discuss other preventive and therapeutic approaches of Maharishi Ayur-Ved, it is appropriate in the context of the primordial sounds of the Ved to discuss briefly one of the most exciting new research projects on Maharishi Ayur-Ved and Maharishi's Vedic Physiology, recently conducted by Dr. Tony Nader. (For now, I will simply describe the main ideas of Dr. Nader's historic discovery. Later on, in Chapters 13 and 14, we will look in detail at the structure of the Vedic literature, and the precise mechanics of how it expresses the sequential unfoldment of the laws of nature from within pure consciousness.)

Through his discussions with Maharishi, Dr. Nader has found that there is an exact, one-to-one correspondence between the various aspects of the Vedic literature and the anatomical structures which together comprise the human brain and nervous system. Thus the Ved is found not only within our consciousness, but throughout our physiology. This remarkable finding is the subject of Dr. Nader's recent book, entitled *Human Physiology: Expression of Ved and the Vedic literature—Modern Science and Ancient Vedic Science Discover the Fabrics of Immortality in the Human Physiology.*

This discovery makes clear that all the creative qualities of consciousness (the Vedic literature), which are the basic unmanifest structure of pure consciousness, are also found in unmanifest form in the different structures of the human brain and nervous system, such as the cortex, hypothalamus, thalamus, etc. The internal mathematical structure of each branch of the Vedic literature precisely corresponds to the internal structure of each of these aspects of the anatomy. Thus, our own physiology is the Ved made manifest.

The primordial sound therapy of Maharishi Ayur-Ved is one practical application of this discovery. Its full implications are vast and far-reaching Through the technologies of Maharishi's Vedic Science and Maharishi Ayur-Ved, especially the Yogic Flying technique of the TM-Sidhi program (described in Chapter 10), all the aspects of the Ved, the Constitution of the Universe—all the aspects of natural law that govern the universe with infinite creativity and infinite organizing power, and without problems or mistakes—become fully awake not only in our consciousness, but throughout our physiology. Then our lives and our health will be supported by the total potential of natural law, free from ,mistakes and problems.

Maharishi Gandharv Ved Therapy and Aroma Therapy

The Maharishi Ayur-Veda Health Center in Lancaster (as well as many other Maharishi Ayur-Ved treatment facilities around the world) offers many therapeutic techniques that, like Primordial Sound therapy, are designed to enliven the body's own inner intelligence and create balance at the finest layers of the physiology of matter. The natural input mechanisms through which these techniques reach the inner network of intelligence are the senses. One such therapy is Maharishi Gandharv Ved music. Vedic texts explain that the melodies of Gandharv Ved, the classical music of the ancient Vedic civilization, are "the melodies of nature"—the intelligence and rhythms of nature expressed in music—and therefore have significant therapeutic value.

Modern science has glimpsed this principle of sounds and melodies at the basis of physical and biological phenomena. In the early 1980s, while studying DNA and molecular evolution, Dr. Susumu Ohno made an interesting discovery. He found that the sequences of nucleotides in DNA that code for life formed patterns similar to those seen in music. Translating these sequences into sheet music, he found that they sounded like the classical music of the Baroque and Romantic periods. The musical patterns within cancer-causing oncogenes sounded somber and funereal, while those within genes that form the lens of the eye sounded airy and playful. While these studies are preliminary and require a degree of extrapolation, they suggest that certain universal patterns underlie human creativity as well as nature's creativity.

The timeless knowledge of Maharishi Ayur-Ved takes a more expanded view: there is order and periodicity in the universe, whether in the motion of the planets or in the genes. The patterns and rhythms of nature are expressions of the fundamental rhythms of the unified field of natural law.

The goal of Maharishi Gandharv Ved therapy, the application of music to health, is to help attune the body to the underlying harmony and orderliness of nature and thereby re-establish physiological balance. Similarly to Primordial Sound therapy, the sounds of Gandharv Ved, according to Maharishi Ayur-Ved, resonate with the body's finest layers of matter and re-enliven the junction point between these structures and the sequence of natural law at their basis in consciousness. The sounds are very soothing, pleasing, and enlivening.

Preliminary research has shown that subjects listening to this music demonstrate a marked reduction in breathing—in some cases with repeated periods of respiratory suspension. These respiratory suspensions were not followed by compensatory hyperventilation, but by low respiration rates. Subjective experiences, especially during these periods of respiratory suspensions, were described in terms of greater inner clarity, wakefulness, and bliss. As mentioned earlier, periods of respiratory suspension have been seen in subjects practicing the Transcendental Meditation technique and have also been correlated with subjective reports of the experience of unbounded consciousness.

The whole purpose of Gandharv Ved therapy is to create happiness and bliss, to nourish the senses, and to clear away imbalances. Gandharv Ved therapy also attunes us to the natural rhythms and cycles of nature. It divides the day into eight important three-hour time periods and prescribes specific types of music to attune us to the laws of nature in each of these periods. These periods are known to be governed by the different doshas; listening to the appropriate Gandharv Ved music at each time is meant to bring balance to the doshas in the physiology.

Another approach of Maharishi Ayur-Ved that uses the senses as a way of influencing the body's intelligence network is Aroma therapy. The patient is treated with certain aromas depending on which doshas or subdoshas are imbalanced. The aromas are usually in the form of oils that are heated to a vapor. The purpose of the aroma is to calm or rebalance the doshas.

There is considerable research on the sense of smell in Western science. Unlike other senses, the sense of smell is not relayed to the brain via one of its central structures (the thalamus), but instead passes directly from the nose to an older part of the brain (the amygdala), which is closely connected to the regulation of emotional reactions. It is clear that certain aromas have the ability to evoke vivid emotional memories.

In terms of Maharishi Ayur-Ved, the purpose of the aroma is again to reset the correct sequential unfoldment of intelligence in the body. It has been proposed that different aromas introduce certain sensory information in the brain, stimulating specific electrophysiological and biochemical pathways that help to remove imbalances and enable the body's inner intelligence to again flow in an orderly and unobstructed manner.

Pranayam

Another way to enter the body's intelligence network is through breath. As part of Maharishi Ayur-Ved, there are specific Vedic breathing exercises, called *pranayam*, which enhance the connection between mind and body and help re-establish balance in the doshas.

Breathing exercises are important therapeutic strategies in many traditional systems of medicine. Recent research suggests how breathing exercises might affect the brain and therefore the entire body. One study measured the influence of breathing exercises on brain waves. The results suggest that patterns of EEG dominance can be affected by the breath.

Measurements show that our breathing follows regular cycles. These nasal cycles involve the rhythmic switching of the airflow from the right to the left nostril over a period of about 90 minutes. When the airflow is predominantly through the right nostril, higher relative amplitudes of EEG activity are found in the left hemisphere, and vice versa.

Further, studies show that the balance of dominance can be shifted by intentionally altering the nasal cycle through pranayam. For example, closing the right nostril and gently breathing through the left nostril causes increased EEG activity in the brain's right hemisphere, and vice versa. One study found that changes in EEG patterns occurred almost instantaneously, and after 10 or 15 seconds a long-lasting shift in EEG dominance occurred. These results suggest that by altering the nasal cycle through specific pranayam exercises, we can alter neurophysiological functioning in the brain.

Almost twenty years ago Nobel laureate Dr. Roger Sperry and his collaborator, Dr. Michael Gazzaniga, found that patients who had undergone surgical separation of the right and left cerebral hemispheres of the brain to prevent the spreading of epileptic seizures showed unusual characteristics. These patients behaved as if each of the two sides of their brains had a mind of its own: the left side saw the world from a more analytical, scientific perspective, while the right side saw the world with a more synthetic, artistic vision. This research inspired other studies into the nature of the brain: over the years, researchers have tried to locate specific control centers in the brain's structure responsible for specific physiological functions. Although the strict division of the brain into right and left is now considered an oversimplification (many processes actually involve whole-brain activity), it has nevertheless proved to be extremely useful.

One of the goals of pranayam is to establish balance in the physiology and psychology. Perhaps by rhythmically altering the nasal cycles, we can establish better integration between the two hemispheres of the brain, between our so-called "scientific" and "artistic" modes of psychological functioning. Since the brain controls all physiological functions, it is reasonable to assume that breathing exercises might affect other parts of the body via the nervous system. In Maharishi Ayur-Ved, these pranayam breathing exercises are used as a general prevention measure and are prescribed for specific conditions depending upon the particular dosh that is imbalanced.

Maharishi Panchakarm Therapy

Maharishi Panchakarm therapy involves purification procedures that are prescribed according to body type. These procedures influence the body's intelligence network through a variety of means, including herbalized oil massages, herbal steam baths, herbal elimination treatments, special eye and nose treatments, and a variety of dietary and behavioral programs.

The panchakarm procedures, according to Maharishi Ayur-Ved, restore balance within the system, specifically balance among the doshas. Ayur-Ved states that the body is permeated by hollow channels called *shrotas* that must be kept open to promote and maintain health. Panchakarm removes any obstruction in the shrotas and thus allows the body's inner intelligence to flow freely. Because of its strengthening and refreshing effects on the mind and body, it is also referred to as "rejuvenation therapy."

Studies show that Maharishi Panchakarm improves mental and physical health and reduces biological age. In one study researchers found that with panchakarm, patients demonstrated improved mental health characterized by significant reductions in negative moods (including anxiety, depression, and fatigue) and increased vigor as compared with control subjects who were given knowledge about Maharishi Ayur-Ved but not the actual treatment. In a similar study, panchakarm subjects showed significant improvements in energy, vitality, well-being, strength, stamina, appetite, digestion, and rejuvenation compared with controls.

Maharishi Panchakarm apparently also affects cholesterol levels. Cholesterol is a topic of great interest to most Americans, and our understanding continues to grow as more research is conducted. We know that, in general, high cholesterol levels are not beneficial to our health; however, we can better understand cholesterol's effects by considering those elements in the blood that transport cholesterol: high- and low-density lipoproteins (HDL and LDL). Higher levels of LDL are associated with increased risk of heart disease. Higher levels of HDL are associated with lower risk of heart disease.

A recent study completed at the University of Freiburg in Germany found a 10% decrease in cholesterol after one to two weeks of Maharishi Panchakarm treatment, compared with no change in a control group. There was also a decrease of 8.7% in LDL. Based on the results of previous studies, the author suggests that Maharishi Panchakarm treatment could reduce the risk of coronary mortality by 17.4%.

These results have been replicated and extended by a recent study in the United States, which found an acute decrease in cholesterol immediately following Maharishi Panchakarm treatment and an increase in HDL levels three months later. In addition, lipid peroxide, a measure of free radical activity (a damaging chemical reaction we will discuss in detail in Chapter 7) was found to rise during panchakarm treatment and then to decrease to lower levels three months later. (The temporary increase might be associated with the purifying nature of this treatment, with the consequent beneficial effect of purification being seen in the eventual lower levels.) Finally, a neuropeptide known as VIP has a number of actions, one of which is increased blood flow in the arteries supplying the heart; VIP was found to increase by 80% three months after treatment.

One further area of research concerns the use of sesame oil, the primary oil used in several treatments. In one of the panchakarm programs known as *abhyang*, herbalized sesame oil is massaged over the entire body with a pressure and speed that depends upon the person's physical condition and body type. Maharishi Ayur-Ved recommends that everybody do a daily sesame oil massage at home. Dr. D. Edwards Smith has been researching the effects of sesame oil. In one procedure known as *gandush*, which involves applying the oil inside the mouth, he found a significant reduction in oral bacterial counts.

Dr. Smith hypothesizes that linoleic acid, which comprises 40% of the fatty acids in sesame oil, may be metabolized into a natural antibacterial agent. Linoleic acid is present in the skin and is known to inhibit the growth of certain pathogenic bacteria. Linoleic acid has also been found to be an anti-inflammatory agent. Dr. Smith and his co-worker Dr. John Salerno have published several research papers on the effects of linoleic acid and sesame oil as preventive chemotherapeutic agents against cancer. They have found that both linoleic acid and sesame oil selectively inhibit the growth of both colon and skin cancer cells *in vitro* (in a cell culture).

The Individual and the Environment

In addition to Gandharv Ved music, Maharishi Ayur-Ved uses several other therapeutic strategies that take into account the relationship of the individual to the environment. One strategy, Maharishi Jyotish, provides a mathematical approach to diagnose and prognosticate disease. Through Maharishi Jyotish the position of any event in the sequential unfolding of natural law can be precisely known; therefore its past, present, and future can be accurately described. A medical condition can thus be perceived with remarkable accuracy in context of its history and prognosis. All that is required is the knowledge of a few key elements.

This principle is a familiar one in Western physiology and medicine. For example, we know that the cells of a human embryo evolve in highly specific ways, due to the information encoded within the cells themselves. At any given stage, we can accurately predict the embryo's development and its reaction to any changes in its environment.

Likewise, through blood tests we can see indicators of potential, nascent, or existing disease. Given these indicators, we can successfully predict what will occur in the future. However, Maharishi Jyotish, instead of relying on gross, external measurements (such as blood samples) used by Western science, relies on precise, mathematically derived descriptions of nature's unfoldment.

In Maharishi Ayur-Ved, Jyotish is used for both prevention and cure. As prevention, it allows the physician to perceive and correct in advance potential imbalances in a patient. As cure, it enables the physician to neutralize negative environmental influences that may be hindering the effective action of other Ayurvedic therapies.

A second strategy, Maharishi Yagya, is the applied aspect of Jyotish. Yagyas are specific Vedic performances that reset the patterns of sequential unfoldment of nature's intelligence in the mind, body, and environment. We can think of these performances as preventive maintenance. Yagyas prevent dangerous conditions before they arise within the physiology of matter by working on the level of the physiology of consciousness.

For individuals with high blood pressure, doctors often prescribe medication and a restricted diet. This is preventive medicine on the level of the physiology of matter. By having these people practice TM regularly, doctors are applying preventive medicine on the level of the physiology of consciousness. In this sense, Transcendental Meditation itself is also a type of yagya.

Because of their broad range of influence, yagyas can be used either as individual or collective health measures. The individual body is made up of a collection of cells; society is like the body in that it is made up of a collection of individuals. Yagyas can be used to help neutralize imbalance in society and thus produce good effects on the overall collective health and quality of life.

What is unique about yagyas is the level of precision and sophistication involved. They are equivalent to the most advanced type of engineering, such as that involved in a flight to the moon. The difference is that a yagya is engineering on the deepest level of natural law—the Constitution of the Universe. This is Vedic engineering: engineering on the level of pure consciousness. Those skilled in the application of yagyas are highly trained in the technologies of consciousness. They must be able to maintain that most silent and unified state of consciousness in their own awareness while they reset the unfoldment of nature's intelligence through these Vedic performances.

In summary, all the approaches of Maharishi Ayur-Ved reconnect the individual's physiology of matter with its source in the physiology of consciousness. Some of the approaches do so by directly enlivening balance from the level of pure consciousness. Other approaches restore balance at the finest level of the physiology of matter—the level of the doshas—using highly individualized treatment and prevention programs based on a thorough understanding of diet, exercise, body types, behavioral tendencies, and biological and seasonal rhythms. This integrated understanding of how to treat our physiology of consciousness and our physiology of matter promises to bring fulfillment to medicine's age-old dream to relieve mankind from disease and suffering.

CHAPTER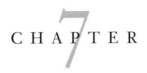

MEDICINAL HERBAL PREPARATIONS

O
N A VISIT SEVERAL YEARS AGO TO THE PHILIPPINES, I MET with one of the top pharmacologists at the University of the Philippines in Manila. She was in charge of a large government project to scientifically evaluate and develop practical procedures for the use of herbal medicines. Quite a large percentage of the rural Filipino population uses herbal medicines, primarily because people cannot afford modern medicines and fear their potential side effects.

In many developing countries the cost of modern medicines is exorbitantly high. For example, I was told that many pharmacies in Brazil act like loan sharks, selling medicine on loan and charging very high interest rates. Another problem is that some powerful drugs we would never consider giving out without a prescription are readily available to people who may not be able to read the instructions.

The pharmacologist in Manila had embarked upon a project to systematically evaluate the most commonly used herbs. It was a very well thought out program, evaluating not only the pharmacological and clinical properties of each herb, but also the best method for the herb's growth, harvest, and conversion into medicine. She explained that in each case they went into great detail in evaluating the herbs and their preparations. For example, an herbal text stated that for one particular medicine, only the top five leaves of a plant should be picked, and only during a particular time and season. The scientists attempted to find out why these instructions were given. As it turned out, when they had isolated what they thought was the most active ingredient, it was found to be most concentrated in the top leaves of the plant, and most abundant at the specified time and season.

Again and again they found that the ancient accounts held important secrets, which—to our loss—have been dismissed as hocus pocus by the average scientist. But this woman was a very good and dedicated scientist, and as a result she was able to take advantage of extremely valuable traditional knowledge. The project was financed primarily by her government, with the long-term goal of reducing both health care costs and the dependence on Western medicine.

This type of project is by no means unique. Many countries have embarked on similar programs. In Kenya I talked with an eminent physiologist at the University of Nairobi who had a longstanding interest in Africa's systems of natural medicine. He pointed out that most of the experts lived in remote areas, and the so-called experts in the cities were often not the true masters of the traditional knowledge at all.

One reason why native medical traditions are being lost is that the knowledge is often passed only from father to son. Unfortunately, many of the younger generation are no longer interested in the old ways; they prefer to move to the cities, drawn by more material Western comforts. As a consequence, the older experts, rather than pass the knowledge of herbal preparations along to just anyone, allow it to die with them. This situation has clearly occurred in many cultures. Compounding it is the loss of cultural integrity caused by conquest and foreign domination. We only have to look at the traditions of Native Americans to realize how easy it is for generations of knowledge to disappear in relatively few years.

Medicinal Herbs in Maharishi Ayur-Ved

One of the great contributions of Maharishi Ayur-Ved is its extensive knowledge of medicinal plants. We are extremely fortunate that Maharishi has gathered the greatest Ayurvedic experts in this area to bring to light once again the knowledge of how these herbs work.

In Maharishi Ayur-Ved, the principle of complementarity holds that the physiologies of plants and animals are upheld by the same patterns of intelligence. Specifically, the sequence of biological information as stored in plants and minerals corresponds to the sequence of biological information in the human physiology. Herbal preparations function, Maharishi explains, like special biological "software" that supplies the essential program to re-establish the order and balance in the source code of the system.

To use another of Maharishi's analogies, the herbal preparations of Maharishi Ayur-Ved act like a set of tuning forks. Just as striking one tuning fork sets an identical one in sympathetic vibration, these herbs resonate in particular frequencies to restore the frequencies of self-interaction associated with proper functioning in the various cells and tissues in the body. To say this a different way, the sequential unfoldment of intelligence in the herbal preparation resonates with the unfoldment of intelligence in the physiology of matter. It resets the correct sequence of unfoldment, removing any distortions that cause obstructions to the flow of intelligence. When these obstructions are removed, the body automatically corrects any imbalances that might lead to disease.

Maharishi Ayur-Ved contains the knowledge of how to use just the right preparations and combinations of very specific plants and minerals to treat a wide variety of disorders. Of particular interest are a group of herbal and mineral preparations known as *rasayanas*. Rasayanas, like the other herbal preparations in Maharishi Ayur-Ved, use this principle of complementarity. However, the function of rasayanas is both preventive as well as curative.

Some of the first studies on rasayanas were conducted at the Massachusetts Institute of Technology and involved a special preparation known as Maharishi Ayur-Ved Bhasma Rasayan. This rasayan was developed by Dr. V. M. Dwivedi, an Ayurvedic physician for over 60 years, who had conducted research for some 30 years and had served on the graduate faculty of India's leading Ayurvedic university. He had worked closely with Maharishi for more than 10 years, and was one of the few remaining individuals in this generation familiar with the highly complex and intricate process of preparing certain longevity-promoting rasayanas. Under his direction and inspiration, several of these special longevity rasayanas were prepared in laboratories in Switzerland and India.

Dr. Tony A. Nader, who is both an M.D. and a Ph.D., studied the effects of Dr. Dwivedi's specially prepared rasayanas. In one experiment, two groups of animals were given a special low-choline, low-methionine, high-fat diet that accelerates the aging process and causes damage to tissues of the kidney, liver, and cardiovascular system. One of two groups was given Dr. Dwivedi's Maharishi Ayur-Ved Bhasma Rasayan. This group showed significantly less kidney and liver damage compared with the control group, which had extensive damage. Biochemical analysis showed insignificant amounts of choline or methionine in the rasayan.

In another study using the same rasayan, Dr. Nader and his co-workers administered a known carcinogen (cancer-causing agent) to two groups of laboratory rats and found that the group given the rasayan had 40% fewer tumors than the group without the rasayan.

Dr. Nader, in collaboration with other researchers, also investigated the effect of Bhasma Rasayan on recovery from neurological damage caused by entorhinal lesions. These lesions are known to lead to severe memory and learning disorders and to impaired cognitive functioning. The study found that animals with lesions responded extremely well when given the rasayan as a dietary supplement. Rasayan-treated animals performed better on learning tasks than did a group given gangliosides, a special group of chemicals that are the most powerful agents known to reduce nerve deficits.

These initial studies give some glimpse into the strikingly beneficial effects of Maharishi Ayur-Ved rasayanas. They were followed by a wide range of studies, particularly on the most important of the rasayanas, known as Maharishi Amrit Kalash.

Maharishi Amrit Kalash

Maharishi has worked closely with several great Ayurvedic experts on herbal preparations. One is Dr. Balraj Maharshi, an advisor on Ayur-Ved to the government of India and perhaps the world's leading expert in *Dravyagun*, the identification and utilization of medicinal plants. He has an extraordinary knowledge of over six thousand plants, many of which are very obscure and located in remote regions of India.

His great experience was illustrated at a conference in Brazil several years ago, which was attended by experts in natural medicine from Chile, Colombia, Bolivia, and other South American countries. Also present was the head of a Brazilian botanical institute located near the Amazon, who had brought with her specimens of many different indigenous plants.

At one point the experts began to examine the plants and exchange knowledge about their medicinal uses. What was striking in this exchange was the very rich and complete knowledge Dr. Balraj brought out. Even though the plants were from an entirely different continent, he was able to bring out several more uses for, and details about many plants than were known by experts from the plants' country of origin.

One of Dr. Balraj's great contributions to Maharishi Ayur-Ved has been his participation in formulating a special herbal rasayan known as Maharishi Amrit Kalash. Rasayanas are designed to act at the most fundamental level of the physiology—the junction point between consciousness and matter. Said to be the "king of rasayanas," Maharishi Amrit Kalash is intended to create balance from this level and establish the basis for fully integrated functioning of mind, body, behavior, and environment. Designed to be taken by all body types, it is probably the only natural food supplement specifically formulated to develop higher states of consciousness.

Maharishi Amrit Kalash comes to us from the long history of the Vedic tradition; its fascinating story parallels the unfoldment of all the areas of Vedic knowledge through the self-interacting dynamics of consciousness. The Vedic literature records that at the dawn of creation, all the forces of nature assembled together to churn the primordial ocean of consciousness. This churning produced a few drops of ambrosia, known as *amrit* (the Sanskrit word for immortality), which was collected in a golden vessel called a *kalash*. This original preparation—the first rasayan—was used to restore the connection between immortal pure consciousness and the physiology to achieve perfection in life.

The formula for Maharishi Amrit Kalash—a compound of precious herbs from the thick forests and Himalayan mountainsides of India— was developed by sages under the leadership of Bhoja Raj, one of the revered kings of India, who distributed it to all his subjects so that they could develop perfect health. As with the entire range of Vedic wisdom, over the course of time the formula and its use became lost to the wider population; but it was closely guarded and handed down by a small number of Ayurvedic physicians in each generation. In modern times, the formula was given to Dr. Balraj.

Dr. Balraj knew that this rasayan was meant to be used on a mass scale for the benefit of society as a whole. He therefore waited for an opportunity to bring it to the world—which came when he met Maharishi Mahesh Yogi. In 1985, Maharishi asked Dr. Balraj, Dr. Dwivedi, and Dr. B. D. Triguna a question similar to one Bhoja Raj had posed to his advisors long ago: What could be done to eliminate disease and suffering and improve the quality of life of everyone in the world? Together with other eminent vaidyas, these three—the world's greatest exponents of Maharishi Ayur-Ved—restored the formula of Amrit Kalash in its completeness so that it could once again be widely available to promote perfect health in the whole population.

Maharishi Amrit Kalash is actually two different compounds composed of 23 herbs: "nectar" (M-4, an herbal fruit concentrate), and "ambrosia" (M-5, in tablet form). In the past few years, these compounds have been the subject of extensive scientific research in different parts of the world, at institutions including the National Institutes of Health and the National Cancer Institute, the Niwa Institute of Immunology in Japan, The Ohio State University College of Medicine, Loyola University Medical School, University of Kansas Medical Center, South Dakota State University, the University of Colorado, Indiana University, SRI International, and the University of California at Irvine.

These studies have shown the rasayan to have many potential benefits for health and longevity. Maharishi Amrit Kalash has been found to:

- inhibit tumor growth (in medical terminology, Maharishi Amrit Kalash is called *anticarcinogenic*—meaning that it both prevented the start (genesis) of cancer and decreased the size of existing tumors (this property is also referred to as *antineoplastic*)
- "scavenge" free radicals (it displayed anti-oxidant properties)
- have a positive influence on known cardiovascular risk factors
- enhance the functioning of immune cells
- promote longevity and have anti-aging effects
- affect cell receptors in the brain and body

In addition, Maharishi Amrit Kalash has been shown to be non-toxic and preventive.

As we will see below, many of the findings are in overlapping areas. One set of positive findings—for example, in cancer—has often suggested effects in other areas (in this case, free radicals and aging); this has stimulated new areas of research and further delineated the wide-ranging effects of this remarkable herbal preparation. Many researchers now feel that the independent research results indicating effects of Maharishi Amrit Kalash on so many diverse areas shows a synergistic effect of the rasayan that probably extends to the whole body. This supports the understanding of Amrit Kalash from Maharishi Ayur-Ved, as a substance that works on the deepest level of intelligence in the body—that level which is all-pervading. Therefore its effects should necessarily be found at all levels of the mind and body.

One eminent researcher who has organized and conducted many studies on Maharishi Amrit Kalash is Hari Sharma, M.D., Professor of Pathology and Director of Cancer Prevention and Natural Products Research at The Ohio State University College of Medicine. Between 1987 and the close of 1991, Dr. Sharma directed ten studies on Maharishi Amrit Kalash involving more than 24 independent researchers at five universities. His pioneering research has inspired scientists around the world to undertake their own investigations. Results of this research have appeared in many respected scientific journals internationally; much of it is summarized in Dr. Sharma's new book, *Freedom from Disease*.

The following sections describe some of the research studies on Maharishi Amrit Kalash, including many of Dr. Sharma's.

Research on Maharishi Amrit Kalash and Cancer

Perhaps the most striking research on Maharishi Amrit Kalash so far concerns its effects on cancer. Several researchers at various institutions have been studying the effects of M-4 and M-5 on different forms of cancer, both in vitro (in test tubes) and in vivo (in laboratory animals). The following section gives a more detailed scientific summary of this research.

Breast cancer. In a series of studies, Dr. Sharma and his co-workers at South Dakota State University and The Ohio State University

College of Medicine investigated the effects of M-4 and M-5 on breast cancer in laboratory animals. In two studies they found that M-4 and M-5 were highly effective in preventing carcinoma of the breast.

One study involved giving animals a potent carcinogen (DMBA). The control group of animals was given DMBA alone. Other groups were given a diet with 0.2% of M-5 at different times, both during and after the administration of DMBA. The goal was to determine at what point in the onset of cancer the rasayan might be most effective.

An "initiation phase" group received M-5 daily for one week before and one week after the carcinogen was administered. A "promotion phase" group was given M-5 daily beginning one week after DMBA was administered and then continuously until the end of the experiment. Finally, there was a third "combined" group that was given M-5 before and after DMBA until the end of the experiment.

After 18 weeks only 25% of animals receiving M-5 during the promotion phase showed tumors, as compared to 66.6% of control animals, who received the carcinogen but not M-5. The investigators concluded that this protection occurred during the promotion phase of carcinogenesis.

Using a similar experimental design, Dr. Sharma and his colleagues examined the effect of a diet supplemented with M-4 on DMBA-induced breast cancer in animals. The effects of M-4 were very striking. In all the groups that received M-4, many fewer animals developed tumors than in the control group. The biggest effect was in the "promotion" phase group—about 88% fewer animals with tumors, compared with the control group.

The number of tumors per animal was also far less in the M-4 groups—85% fewer tumors per animal were observed in both the promotion and combined groups, compared with the control animals. Control animals that had already developed fully formed tumors were then administered M-4 for a period of four weeks; in 60% of the animals, tumors smaller than a critical size either shrank or disappeared entirely. Repeat experiments using a combination of M-4 and M-5 confirmed the findings indicating prevention of DMBA-induced breast cancer.

Lung cancer. In a study on lung cancer, Dr. Vimal Patel and his colleagues at the medical schools of Indiana University and Ohio State studied the effects of M-4 on the process of cancer metastasis (the spread of tumor cells to distant organs). They found that animals with advanced Lewis lung cancer, a model of aggressive metastasizing cancer of the lung, showed a 45–65% reduction in both the size and number of metastatic lung cancer nodules when fed M-4 in their diet.

Neuroblastoma. Dr. Kedar Prasad, Director of the Center for Vitamin and Cancer Research at the Health Sciences Center, University of Colorado, researched the effects of M-5 on neuroblastoma cells (a form of neurological cancer, often found in children, that is considered especially difficult to treat). Treatment for neuroblastoma with conventional therapies can generate severe side-effects.

Malignant neuroblastoma cells typically multiply uncontrollably. Using cell cultures, Dr. Prasad found that M-5 caused "differentiation" of neuroblastoma cells into mature, normal-like neuronal cells. That is, after exposure to M-5, neuroblastoma cells showed several signs of normality, including stoppage of rampant growth, larger cell bodies, and the formation of well-developed finger-like projections (dendrites). Their biochemical functioning also appeared normal: there was increased production of enzymes normally produced by healthy cells.

Thus, the cancerous cells were transformed into cells with normal shape and behavior, as if M-5 had restored their molecular memory of how to function as healthy cells. Maharishi Amrit Kalash is reportedly one of the few non-toxic agents able to produce such an effect; several other agents which produce differentiation are known to be toxic.

In addition, the continued presence of M-5 in the culture prevented rapid degeneration of the improved cells, giving further evidence of M-5's protective effect.

Skin cancer. Dr. Brian Johnston and his colleagues at SRI International (formerly Stanford Research Institute) studied the therapeutic value of M-5 against DMBA-induced papilloma, a form of skin cancer. Mice that were fed M-5 in their diet had consistently and significantly lower mortality over the course of the experiment: they showed 75% survival, compared with 31% survival in the control group. The SRI research team reports that the findings indicate the M-5 had a significant therapeutic effect.

Inhibiting cell transformation. In research supported by the National Cancer Institute (NCI), Julia T. Arnold and her colleagues at ManTech Environmental Technology in North Carolina and at NCI in Bethesda, Maryland, studied the effect in vitro of extracts of M-4 and M-5 on human tumor cells and on animal tracheal cells to which a cancer-causing agent had been added. Extracts of M-4 inhibited transformation of healthy cells into cancer cells in both the animal and human cell cultures. An aqueous (water-based) extract of M-5 inhibited transformation of the animal tracheal cell cultures.

Taken together, the results of all these studies suggest that Maharishi Amrit Kalash may have great value in the prevention and treatment of cancer. In 1990, the National Cancer Institute included M-4 and M-5 on its list of potential chemopreventive agents.

A wide-ranging research effort is currently in progress to continue and broaden the investigation of Maharishi Amrit Kalash. To determine its cancer prevention properties, NCI is funding a series of in vitro studies on Amrit Kalash at SRI International, IITRI at the University of Chicago, and at ManTech in North Carolina. Dr. Sharma's team that studied breast cancer at South Dakota State and Ohio State is preparing a series of new studies (a) to examine the effect of M-4 and M-5 on other forms of cancer; (b) to examine their possible effects on cancers in human subjects; and (c) to identify their mechanisms of action.

Scavenging Free Radicals

The cancer studies on Maharishi Amrit Kalash led some researchers to suspect that its cancer-inhibiting properties might be tied to an effect on free radicals. What are free radicals? They are highly reactive, electrochemically unstable atoms and molecules.

The structure of these molecules, particularly their unpaired outer electrons, is what makes them so unstable and highly reactive. We can visualize these outer electrons as spinning at great velocities around the core of an atom or molecule in imaginary shells or orbits. Most stable chemical compounds contain two paired electrons in these shells. A free radical is characterized by the presence of an unpaired single electron in its outer shell, causing a tendency to react with other molecules. The type of reaction that occurs when a free radical comes in contact with other molecules is usually extremely damaging. It can be so damaging that it causes other free-radical reactions, setting off a chain reaction.

Most free radicals, unlike foreign invaders such as bacteria or viruses, are produced as a normal part of the body's use of oxygen. The use of oxygen gives us the enormous advantage of being able to harness and metabolize energy from our environment. In fact, oxygen use is essential to higher forms of life; yet it also brings with it potential damages due to the free radicals inevitably created during cellular metabolism. Free radicals occur in humans, animals, plants, the atmosphere, and many chemical systems. There are many different kinds, including lipid peroxides and superoxide.

The body's immune system needs free radicals to defend itself from the onslaughts of bacteria and viruses. However, if too many free radicals are generated, they start to attack the body: they damage DNA and cause usually-benign chemicals in the body to become toxic.

Many aspects of modern life, such as pollution (including cigarette smoke), improper diet, and stress are known to contribute to the uncontrolled formation of free radicals, which can then initiate chain reactions capable of causing extensive damage to normal cells and tissues. Other factors known to contribute to excess free radical production include excessive radiation from the sun or tanning lamps, agricultural chemicals, processed foods (especially meat), coffee, overexertion in muscular activity, alcohol consumption, exposure to many industrial solvents, X-rays, exhaust fumes, ozone, and anti-cancer treatments such as radiation and chemotherapy.

Over the past few years, free radicals have received considerable scientific attention, owing to their having been identified in various disease states and in aging. (For example, the Free Radical Society was established at the National Institutes of Health in 1988; the International Society for Free Radical Research has also been established.)

Free radicals have been implicated in the development of approximately 80% of diseases and environmental toxicities, including atherosclerosis, rheumatoid arthritis, cancer, cataracts, diabetes, inflammatory bowel disease, emphysema, Alzheimer's disease, depression of the immune system, side-effects of radiation, and degenerative processes associated with aging. Also, the toxic effects associated with certain chemicals and drugs are reported to be linked to free radical generation and lipid peroxidation. (The havoc wrought by free radicals is not confined to living systems: when rust slowly eats away at a car, that process is also mediated by free radicals.

How can the body protect itself against the ravages of free radicals?

Medical science has spent millions of dollars attempting to find effective ways to "scavenge," or remove them. A number of naturally occurring substances are known to be anti–free radical agents: for example, alpha tocopherol (vitamin E), tannic acid, flavonoids, catechin, flavoproteins, polyphenols, ascorbic acid (vitamin C), riboflavin (vitamin B_2), and beta carotene. It also turns out that the body produces its own powerful natural free radical scavengers, including an enzyme called superoxide dismutase (SOD).

Some researchers have "purified" SOD—that is, they have isolated it from cells so that it can be administered as a treatment. However, because the body breaks down proteins such as SOD in the digestive system and blood stream, SOD is not assimilated through the gastrointestinal tract and is short-lived outside of living cells. Thus it isn't useful to give purified SOD orally (in fact, taking too much can actually generate free radicals). Injections of SOD have been tried, but the effects of these last only a short time (the "half-life" of SOD in blood is only six minutes). SOD has been useful clinically in some acute circumstances, but for long-term prevention of the effects of free radicals, SOD injections are an impractical form of treatment.

Dr. Yukie Niwa, one of the world's leading immunologists, has been studying free radicals for over 20 years at the Niwa Institute in Japan. Dr. Niwa has tested over 500 compounds for their free radical–scavenging effects. He became interested in Maharishi Amrit Kalash as a result of Dr. Sharma's research, and conducted in vitro research with biochemical systems and human white blood cells, to investigate M-4 and M-5 as potential free radical scavengers.

Free radical research. In one series of tests conducted on animals and humans, Dr. Niwa looked at the ability of Amrit Kalash to influence inflammation response. Free radicals are released during the inflammation response by certain immune cells (such as neutrophils) to fight viruses and bacteria. Dr. Niwa measured the activity of the neutrophils and the amount of free radicals generated. When M-4 and M-5 were administered, they decreased both the activity of the neutrophils and the amount of free radicals.

Other studies have investigated Maharishi Amrit Kalash and free radicals. Dr. Sharma's findings on preventing and reversing chemically induced breast cancer prompted Dr. Jeremy Fields and his colleagues at Loyola University Medical School and the Hines V.A. Hospital in Illinois to test their hypothesis that Amrit Kalash might contain one or more scavengers of particular free radicals. In their studies, the rasayan efficiently scavenged free radicals produced by white blood cells, without damaging the cells' structure or function.

Fields' group was testing Maharishi Amrit Kalash against superoxide anions, a type of oxygen free radical produced by human white blood cells. Amrit Kalash scavenged 100% of the superoxide anions—it was as competent as SOD and as potent, milligram for milligram, at scavenging them. Another free radical generated by white blood cells is hypochlorous acid (HOCl), which may be even more directly involved in tissue injury. In vitro, at similar concentrations of Amrit Kalash, HOCl was also scavenged.

In our laboratories at MIU, M-4 and M-5 were also found to be effective scavengers of superoxide radicals. Aqueous extracts of M-4 and M-5 scavenged, respectively, 96% and 98% of the superoxide radicals generated in an enzymatic system similar to that used by Dr. Niwa and Dr. Fields.

Lipid peroxides. One class of oxygen free radicals includes lipid peroxides. Lipids (fats) are a category of biomolecules, along with proteins, that make up cell walls. Free radicals are not usually long-lived, but they can latch onto these lipids and transform them into lipid peroxides (such as those found in rancid oils)—potent oxygen radicals that can cause damage to arterial linings and thus contribute to heart disease. Several studies have explored the effects of Maharishi Amrit Kalash on reducing lipid peroxides.

Working with Dr. Sharma, Dr. C. Dwivedi and his co-workers at South Dakota State University found that extracts of both M-4 and M-5 significantly reduced lipid peroxide levels in test tube systems, using animal subjects. An aqueous extract of M-4 was the most effective—it inhibited lipid peroxidation by approximately 50%.

In a study described below on platelet aggregation in rabbits on high cholesterol diets, Dr. Sharma and a colleague also found that lipid peroxides in blood plasma and liver cells were significantly lower in the rabbits whose diets included M-4.

In another study, Dr. Sharma and his colleagues at Ohio State studied the ability of Maharishi Amrit Kalash to inhibit LDL oxidation in solution. (This refers to the oxidation of lipids in low-density lipoproteins circulating in the blood.) They compared M-4 and M-5 (as well as other Maharishi Ayur-Ved preparations) to vitamin C and to probucol, a drug commonly used to prevent oxidation of lipids.

They found that very small concentrations of M-4 and M-5 reduced lipid peroxidation—the concentrations were approximately 9,000 times less (M-4) and 100,000 times less (M-5) than the amount of probucol needed to produce the same percent reduction. More research needs to be done to fully explore this area, but these initial findings are intriguing.

Industrial solvents. Over two million workers in the United States are exposed daily to the damaging effects of the industrial solvent toluene. In a study on the protective effects of Maharishi Amrit Kalash against toluene, Dr. Stephen Bondy of the University of California at Irvine found that animals pre-treated for three days with M-5 and then exposed to toluene showed no evidence of the usual toluene-induced free radical damage.

How does MAK eliminate free radicals? The exact composition of its various ingredients is not fully known, but analysis has shown that it contains many of the known natural anti–free radical agents listed above. (Dr. Sharma and his co-workers suggest that it would be interesting to determine whether the M-4 and M-5 components necessary for its anti-oxidant properties are the same as those responsible for its anti-cancer effects.) It has also been suggested that M-4 and M-5 may modulate free radical processes by "quenching" (subduing) free radicals or by diverting electrons away from the biological pathway leading to lipid peroxide formation.

A number of researchers, including Dr. Niwa, feel that the unusual ability of Maharishi Amrit Kalash to scavenge free radicals and lipid peroxides explains its diverse effects on cancer, cardiovascular risk factors, and central nervous system activity

Dr. Sharma concurs, seeing M-4 and M-5 as "powerful antioxidants"—having a beneficial effect on a wide range of physiological processes. The consistently good research results in both animals and humans have prompted him to speculate on the possible role of M-4 and M-5 in preventing cancer. "Why does everyone not get cancer?" he asks. "Some people apparently have a natural ability to produce antioxidants and limit free radicals." As he points out, however, the research findings suggest that even for people who seem to produce an adequate supply of antioxidants when they are healthy and living in a healthy environment, M-4 and M-5 may enhance protective mechanisms when those people are exposed to excessive free radicals.

Effects on Cardiovascular Disease:
Reduced Platelet Aggregation

Dr. Sharma has considered carefully the interdependent factors that influence the development of cardiovascular disease. Several of his studies, including the earliest ones he did on Maharishi Amrit Kalash, investigated the effects of M-4 or M-5 on these factors, and he has found the rasayan to have a beneficial influence on all of them.

In the context of discussing free radicals, we have described the studies on M-4 and M-5 in scavenging lipid peroxides. Because lipid peroxides are known to damage artery linings, these findings obviously may have important implications for cardiovascular health.

Another important factor known to contribute to cardiovascular disease is platelet aggregation. Platelets are small cell fragments that circulate in the blood. They tend to clump together and promote clot formation at the site of any injury to the blood vessels. Platelet aggregation either directly or indirectly contributes to a blockage of the arteries to the heart, and is therefore a prime cause of most heart attacks. It plays a significant role in atherosclerosis (hardening of the arteries), a major cardiovascular disorder.

Platelet Aggregation. In one study, Dr. Sharma and his co-workers at Ohio State tested the effect of M-5 in vitro on the action of a number of factors known to cause platelet aggregation. First, in plasma obtained from normal, healthy subjects, they induced platelet aggregation by arachidonic acid, collagen, epinephrine, and ADP. When an extract of M-5 was added to the plasma in the test tube, it dramatically inhibited platelet aggregation: the M-5 decreased platelet aggregation caused by arachidonic acid, epinephrine, and collagen, and fully reversed the aggregation caused by ADP. In a platelet-rich whole blood solution, they found that the extract of M-5 inhibited platelet aggregation caused by collagen and ADP.

These results are of particular interest since a recent large study showed that aspirin taken daily reduced the incidence of heart attacks by 40%. The principle mechanism of aspirin is to reduce platelet aggregation, although aspirin has other unfortunate side effects, including a slight increase in the incidence of certain types of strokes. The mechanism of the action of Maharishi Amrit Kalash seems to be different from that of aspirin, and Amrit Kalash apparently has no harmful side effects. Researchers have continued to test its potential application in both the prevention and treatment of various types of heart disease.

Dr. Sharma and an Ohio State colleague also studied the effect of Maharishi Amrit Kalash on platelet aggregation in rabbits. In their study, rabbits were given a high (1%) cholesterol diet. When M-4 was given along with the high cholesterol diet, the platelet aggregation caused by ADP and collagen was significantly lower in M-4 treated animals than in the controls.

Dr. Sharma feels that the retardation of platelet aggregation by Maharishi Amrit Kalash may be very useful in cardiovascular disorders where prevention of platelet aggregation is of benefit to the patients.

Maharishi Amrit Kalash attacks what are emerging as the underlying causes of atherosclerosis: it is a highly effective scavenger of free radicals, including the lipid peroxides that contribute to hardening of the arteries; it decreases clotting of platelets, further reducing the danger of atherosclerosis; and it is free of harmful side effects. Considering these cardiovascular risk factors, Maharishi Amrit Kalash may come out ahead of other potential treatments.

Enhancement of Immune Function

Another possible mechanism suggested for the effects of Maharishi Amrit Kalash on disease prevention is enhancement of the functioning of the immune system. Increased resistance to disease and infection is one of the effects that Maharishi Ayur-Ved predicts for Maharishi Amrit Kalash. It is well known that excessive and inappropriate immune response is associated with hay fever and rheumatoid arthritis. In addition to reducing the excessive immune response associated with hay fever (described below), research has found that Maharishi Amrit Kalash strengthens the appropriate immune response associated with preventing contagious diseases and infections.

A group of investigators, including Dr. Sharma, from the medical schools of the University of Kansas, Indiana University, and Ohio State noted that Amrit Kalash enhanced the activity of immune system lymphocytes taken from the spleen. These cells are believed to be important not only in protecting against certain types of cancer, but also in preventing infectious diseases.

Immune Studies. In their first study, a group of animals given M-5 for 20 days was compared with a control group not given M-5. After 10 days, all the animals were injected with ovalbumin, an antigen (foreign substance) that stimulates the immune system. After 21 days, immune system cells removed from the spleen were examined for "lymphocyte proliferation"—the rapid multiplication of the immune cells in response to the antigen. Lymphocyte proliferation in the M-5 animals was twice that of the control group at the lowest ovalbumin concentration; at the highest dose of ovalbumin, it was 159% that of the controls.

A subsequent and far more extensive in vitro and in vivo study without ovalbumin immunization showed that the in vitro proliferation of splenic lymphocytes from animals taking M-5 for 10 days was greater than that of control cells. And the response of cells from the group taking M-5 for 20 days was more than twice as great as the response of control cells. There was a very striking increase in the proliferative activity of the immune cells, and the effect persisted for 15 days after the discontinuation of M-5 administration. The results indicate that when the immune system is challenged, the effect of M-5 is to markedly strengthen the immune response.

The researchers suggest that enhanced immune response may be responsible not only for the anti-cancer results found in other research, but also for a decrease in allergic symptoms that has been found in humans. Several years ago a study by Dr. Jay Glaser tested the effect of Maharishi Amrit Kalash on seasonal allergy symptoms. A prospective, double-blind, and placebo-controlled trial was conducted during the spring allergy season. The symptoms of allergy were measured by a daily diary developed at Johns Hopkins, one of the most commonly used measures of allergy patients' response to intervention.

Forty-six allergy sufferers were pair-matched with controls by age, gender, medications used, and severity of symptoms, then randomly assigned to take either M-5 twice daily or a placebo. Those taking M-5 had significantly lower allergy symptoms during three of the four weeks of the study. The most significant differences occurred during the first week, during which both the highest pollen count and greatest symptom severity were recorded.

As with other immune studies described above, Dr. Glaser suggests that Maharishi Amrit Kalash functions as an immune modulator not simply by enhancing the immune response, but by reducing the inappropriate response of the immune system to non-threatening stimuli such as pollen, thus conserving immune reserve and heightening immune sensitivity and responsivity. These effects, he says, could be acting on many different levels of the immune system: humoral, cellular, or even on immune regulators such as steroids and other factors. The studies support this hypothesis, since M-5 appears both to strengthen some aspects of the immune system and to suppress others.

Effects on Cell Receptors: Implications for Mental Health

Another interesting and promising area of research on Maharishi Amrit Kalash involves its effects on cell receptors. Dr. Sharma and his co-workers studied the effects of M-5 on animal brain opioid receptors.

Most drugs act via receptors in the cell membrane. For years, researchers have been investigating those receptors through which opioid drugs (such as morphine) act. As I mentioned in the Overview at the beginning of the book, the body produces its own internal (endogenous) opioids—the endorphins and enkephalins. These chemicals are often produced during stress or injury and act as natural painkillers. They also have been reported to modulate immune functions and to produce the feeling of euphoria.

Dr. Sharma found that M-5 interacted with the receptors for the endorphins and enkephalins. He suggests that Maharishi Amrit Kalash could affect the same receptors in humans, and thus influence our moods and our mental health. Amrit Kalash could therefore be useful in counteracting opioid addiction and helping patients with depression.

On the basis of these results, Dr. Sharma and his colleagues at Ohio State conducted a study on the effects of Maharishi Amrit Kalash on depression. They administered a standard questionnaire to people who had been taking Amrit Kalash from one to three months. Responses indicated that in normal subjects, M-5 may reduce depression and improve mental health.

A study done in our own laboratory at MIU has shown the effects of M-5 on the imipramine receptor. Imipramine is one of the major drugs given for depression. Its precise actions are not well understood, but it binds strongly to a site on cell membranes and increases the activity of a well-studied neurotransmitter called serotonin. Low serotonin–related activity has been associated with depression and many other mental health problems. In human white blood cells, M-5 has an effect similar to imipramine in its interaction with serotonin in platelets, thus suggesting its role in positively influencing mood and mental health.

At a conference in Washington, D.C., several years ago, Dr. Sharma suggested that many of the benefits of Maharishi Amrit Kalash could be due to its ability to affect the cell receptors. "The cell receptors are so intelligent," he said. "They know the changing phases of the sun, and other delicate changes which operate in nature. . . . The receptors receive information, interpret information correctly, and apply information to maintain perfect harmony and balance in the body. What maintains the normal functioning of these receptors? The physiology of the receptor is based on what we eat, what we drink, what we breathe, what we take in, and the influences of the environment and the surroundings that we live in.

"Maharishi Ayur-Ved makes sure our receptors are physiologically active, integrated, and functioning normally. Maharishi Amrit Kalash has the remarkable ability to delicately adjust those receptors such that disease is eliminated and a state of perfect balance is established."

Effects on Life Span, Aging, and Health

One of the free radical studies described above, by Dr. Fields and his colleagues, was conducted in the context of a larger conceptual framework of factors involved in aging. Dr. Fields notes that although aging is a concept that is not clearly defined, it can be seen as a process that increases susceptibility to disease and dysfunction. Any intervention that retarded or reversed this process could be expected to decrease disease, improve human function, and thereby increase quality of life and survival time.

Dr. Fields wanted to test the substantial anti-aging properties that Maharishi Ayur-Ved predicts for Maharishi Amrit Kalash. He and his colleagues therefore studied its effects on aging and related parameters. In a finding directly related to aging, they found that Maharishi Amrit Kalash (M-4 and M-5) extended the life span of mice and fruit flies. The experimental groups receiving M-4 and M-5 as supplements lived significantly longer than the controls, which were fed a standard diet— an average of 20% longer for the mice and over 70% longer for the fruit flies.

According to Dr. Fields, Dr. Sharma's findings on the cancer-preventing effects of Maharishi Amrit Kalash also suggest an anti-aging effect, whose mechanisms may include scavenging of reactive oxygen metabolites (ROM) by low molecular weight anti-oxidants. Dr. Fields' findings on free radicals, described above, lend further weight to this idea.

Clinical research has also investigated age-related factors in human beings. A study by Dr. Paul Gelderloos and his colleagues investigated the effects of M-5 on a visual discrimination task closely related with aging. Forty-eight men over 35 years of age participated in the study and were randomly assigned to two groups, one that took M-5 for six weeks, and a control group that took a closely matched placebo. The M-5 group improved significantly more than the controls in their performance of this task. Successful performance apparently requires an unrestricted flow of attention as well as focused concentration, which involve several different areas of the brain; the researchers suggest that Maharishi Amrit Kalash may therefore influence the nervous system as a whole. They suggest that it may enhance the capacity of attention and alertness, and reverse some of the decline in cognitive abilities that comes as a result of aging.

Several clinical studies with human subjects have examined the effects of Maharishi Amrit Kalash on overall health.

A recent cross-sectional survey of 659 men and women who had been taking M-4 and M-5 an average of 22 months reported substantial benefits in both mental and physical health. The subjects' average age was 41. The results showed that:

- 87% reported increased resistance to illness;
- 83% experienced increased tranquility and calm; 80% reported increased mental clarity and emotional balance;
- 94% of subjects with previous discomforts reported a reduction in frequency of colds, 81% a reduction in hay fever, 87% a reduction in constipation, and 78% a reduction in headaches;
- 84% of women reported reduction of premenstrual syndrome (PMS);
- 84% experienced greater happiness.

Blood chemical analysis and a complete blood profile of 84 people who had been taking Maharishi Amrit Kalash regularly for at least six months and up to four years disclosed no evidence of toxicity or physiological harm. The researchers concluded from blood analysis and self reports that Amrit Kalash may be a useful therapeutic adjunct, a helpful preventive agent, and a safe candidate for clinical trials.

New Directions for Research

As we have seen, researchers are seeking to document and understand not only the seemingly endless benefits of Maharishi Amrit Kalash on many areas of the body, but also some of the possible mechanisms responsible for its range of good effects. More research is necessary to precisely pinpoint these mechanisms; so far, free radicals, enhancement of immune function, and cell receptors are good candidates. It is likely that no one mechanism is completely responsible, but that they all work together to produce such a wide variety of effects.

Research is continuing—in fact, proliferating—in many areas. In progress are studies on atherosclerosis, aging, human DNA repair, reduction of oxidative stress (free radicals), cancer of the colon and of the liver, and protection against cardiac toxicity. A series of tests on Maharishi Amrit Kalash has been funded by the National Cancer Institute at several U.S. research institutions, including further research projects on skin, breast, human lung, and trachial cancer cells, as well as on the biological mechanisms underlying its ability to prevent cancer.

As more research is conducted and published, knowledge of and interest in Maharishi Amrit Kalash spreads further into the medical and scientific community around the world. The focused attention and deep analytical thinking of an increasing number of experts is being drawn to investigate and fully comprehend all the valuable properties of this extraordinary substance, which shows such great promise for the health of the world.

The FDA and Herbal Preparations

If these herbal preparations have such good effects on health, why haven't they been used before in the West? The most important reason is that the traditional knowledge of herbs was lost—even in India. Another very important factor is the U.S. Food and Drug Administration (FDA). In the United States, FDA regulations require an enormous amount of scientific investigation to be completed before any new drug or preparation can be prescribed for a specific disorder.

The caution with modern drugs is well-founded. We only have to remember the disastrous results with the premature use of drugs such as thalidomide, which caused widespread fetal abnormalities, to welcome the FDA's many regulations. It is currently estimated that to complete the necessary steps for testing a new drug, a pharmaceutical company must spend, over a five- to twelve-year period, over $200 million. Why does it cost so much? A battery of tests with different species of animals, ranging from rats to primates, must be done. Long-term clinical trials in humans must demonstrate not only that the drug has specific effects for a specific disease, but more importantly that its side effects are thoroughly known.

It is unfortunate, however, that in the United States the same regulations also apply to herbal medicine. There is a "grandfather" clause that allows preparations used for a long time in this country with no serious side effects to bypass all the regulations. Thus certain herbal tonics and the entire system of homeopathic medicine are overlooked. However, this clause does not apply to herbal preparations used for thousands of years in other countries, such as China and India. Although these preparations produce many verifiable health benefits without side effects, they are not permissible as prescription drugs. Therefore, getting an herbal medicine officially approved to treat a specific disease requires spending almost $200 million.

Many commonly used drugs have been derived from plants. For example, the active ingredient in aspirin is a synthetic derivative of a compound present in the bark of the willow tree. One of the most powerful drugs used in treating heart attacks, digitalis, was derived from the flowering plant foxglove, and the chemotherapeutic agent vincristine comes from the Madagascar periwinkle.

Unfortunately, only a fraction of the knowledge of medicinal plants has ever been utilized. In fact, at a lecture I gave in Egypt some years ago to a conference of physicians, it was pointed out that what had survived from the great systems of herbal medicine were mostly not the useful ingredients, but rather the potentially harmful ones—such as opium, cocaine, caffeine, and nicotine—considered by most pharmacologists as poisons.

Another serious roadblock to their acceptance is that most preparations of herbal medicine involve whole plants or many plants, as well as minerals. Drug companies are generally reluctant to develop and patent such complex preparations. Their primary approach is to isolate and then patent an active ingredient or some similar synthetic product, thus insuring the protection of their multi-million dollar investment.

While financially logical, this approach contains a great medical fallacy. Even in simple herbal preparations there is usually more than one active chemical ingredient. Although one chemical may be the most important for producing the medicinal effect, the other ingredients often serve to counteract any possible side effects. This is the principle of synergy in Maharishi Ayur-Ved. In contrast, most modern drugs contain only one active ingredient. It almost always produces side effects. Thus the whole plant or herbal preparation is more holistic and safer than a modern drug. When we isolate the active ingredient, we take some partial knowledge from the plant but lose its holistic wisdom.

The Future of Traditional Medicine

Many herbs, tonics, various kinds of Chinese medicine, and the like abound in certain kinds of health food stores. Proponents sometimes make what the FDA considers to be illegal and often untrue claims. I have spoken directly with several top FDA officials who said quite frankly that they just don't have the personnel to enforce all of the agency's regulations. Some countries, such as Switzerland, have altered their laws so medical officials can grant licenses to produce and sell beneficial herbal compounds as drugs with specific claims.

The whole picture becomes really complicated when we realize that in many systems of traditional medicine, certain common foods are considered drugs because they can help cure very specific conditions. Should the FDA regulate honey or milk since they are said in the traditional system of Indian medicine to be good for curing certain diseases? Hardly. But there must eventually be a change in our FDA laws, and it probably will have to be initiated from the top.

When former President Nixon first visited China, he became very interested in Chinese medicine, specifically in acupuncture. A directive came from the president's office to the National Institutes of Health to look into traditional Chinese medicine, and suddenly a lot of money was available for research in this area. While traditional Chinese medicine is still a long way from receiving blanket approval, certain procedures such as acupuncture can now be officially practiced in many states as long as the technician is licensed by an approved agency.

I have visited China several times. I have spoken with scientists, given lectures at universities and at the Colleges of Traditional Medicine, and taken part in a lively private meeting with the Minister of Health. Chinese traditional medicine includes meditation, acupuncture, herbal medicines, holistic diets, breathing techniques, longevity treatments, and an enormous variety of exercise, including the martial arts. Traditional medicine is part of the essential fabric of life in China. In the early morning many hundreds of people, including the very elderly, can be seen exercising and meditating in parks, squares, and on rooftops. Herbal medicines are everywhere; one especially finds preparations formulated to promote the extension of life. From early childhood on, the Chinese know that a certain food will produce a hot or cold effect on the body, and that disease is caused by an imbalance in the underlying forces of yin and yang. When people go to the hospital, they now have a choice of Western or traditional Chinese medical treatment.

A number of international organizations, such as the World Health Organization, encourage the revival of traditional systems of medicine. One of the most useful programs that has been developed is the collection onto one large computer database of all research done on the different herbs. This database, known as Napralert, or Natural Products Alert, is located at the University of Illinois in Chicago and provides free information for developing countries.

Unfortunately, so much knowledge in many of these traditional systems of medicine has been lost over time, especially with the current emphasis on modern medicine. It is essential that there be a rapid revitalization of traditional systems of medicine in all countries. With its comprehensive approach, Maharishi Ayur-Ved can help restore each system of traditional medicine to its full potential.

For example, the extensive knowledge contained in Maharishi Ayur-Ved about plants and mineral preparations should be a great resource in rediscovering the uses of medicinal plants in each country. The materia medica of Ayur-Ved is very complete. Using it as a basis for comparison will ensure that the materia medica for all systems of traditional medicine become more complete and comprehensive.

Another important aspect of the revival of traditional medical systems will be to encourage scientists at established universities to conduct research on the numerous medicinal plants.

Plants are one of our least expensive and yet potentially most important resources for the improvement of health. One of the most serious problems today is the preservation of invaluable plant materials in every country that are on the verge of becoming extinct. Whole species of medicinal plants are being totally eliminated as forests and jungles are claimed for agricultural purposes. The medicinal plants of every country offer the potential for greatly reducing health care costs. If this resource is destroyed, it will be a loss not only to the people and economy of the country, but also to the world.

Maharishi Ayur-Ved is helping to educate scientists and health care professionals about the invaluable potential of medicinal plants. It is not an easy process, since we have come to depend almost completely upon synthetic drugs—even with their host of unwanted side effects. The benefits of medicinal plants, however, are vast: drastic reductions of health care costs; elimination of many of the abhorrent side effects of modern drugs; the offer of new treatments, as well as new methods of prevention, for diseases considered incurable by modern medicine; and most of all the natural promotion of health and longevity.

8

AGING AND LIFE EXTENSION: THE SEARCH FOR LONGEVITY

I REMEMBER ONE OF THE FIRST LECTURES I EVER HEARD MAHA-rishi give, almost 30 years ago in Los Angeles. In that talk he described an entirely new level of physiological functioning. "About immortality on the physical level," he said, ". . . when the mind experiences finer realms of thought during meditation, then the metabolism is reduced. As the metabolism is reduced, the activity of the mind becomes finer and finer, and the metabolism becomes further reduced. The mind transcends and gets to that state of transcendental consciousness. Simultaneously the body, the mind, the entire functioning of the inner machinery, the whole metabolic rate comes to zero.

"When this happens, the physical structure of the nervous system comes to a state where it knows no action . . . it remains lively, yet without activity. This is that state where there is no decay. . . . Physical decay comes through activity. Cessation of activity results in cessation of the decaying process. . . . The field of activity means the field of change, means the field of death, to be permeated, to be supported, to go hand in hand with that which never changes: imperishable, absolute Being [pure consciousness], eternal silence."

Maharishi explained that this teaching of immortality was the greatest blessing of the Vedic tradition. It teaches us how to act while remaining non-acting; how to be in the field of relative, temporary existence, yet established in that field of eternal existence, never-changing Being. He said, "Behave in the temporary, remain in the permanent, everlasting, eternal life—this is the teaching of the Vedas."

These words had an enormous impact on both my personal life and my professional career. They inspired me to enter the field of physiology. They were the basis for my doctoral thesis and for subsequent research on transcendental consciousness and its effects on the aging process. They gave me a different perspective from which to view the body. I began to see the physiology of consciousness and the physiology of matter as one integrated network, which, when fully enlivened, has enormous potential benefit for health and longevity.

Immortality

For most scientists, as indeed for most people, the word immortality has an almost fanciful, story-book connotation, something rarely mentioned because of its impractical nature. In the discipline of physiology, what is most apparent is death and change. Nothing lives forever. Trillions of organisms grow and die every second. Innumerable physical structures are created and destroyed. Yet the element of non-change is implicit in biological organisms. From the broad perspective of biological evolution—in the perpetuation of a species—the whole purpose of life indeed seems to be directed towards immortality.

For most organisms, immortality means the continuity of their DNA. Their entire lives are designed around the single function of reproduction. Perhaps there is no better example of this phenomenon than in the life of the Pacific Northwest salmon. Hatched in inland streams, baby salmon migrate to the sea. Once they reach maturity they undergo an epic journey to return to their original spawning grounds and ensure the "immortality" of their species.

The ability of certain living creatures to maintain the existence of their species over millions of years is a remarkable feat of nature. Even man's greatest monuments, such as the pyramids of Egypt, created by highly developed civilizations to record and glorify their power, have slowly eroded, and continue to crumble away into fine grains of sand. It is inevitable that over time the order of a physical system will tend to dissipate, to mix with other elements of the environment. Yet many of the organisms that live in the cracks of decaying pyramids and in the surrounding sand existed as species long before the civilizations that built those monuments were born. These organisms will continue to exist for centuries to come. Perhaps they will find their way onto a spacecraft someday and be carried to other hospitable planets where they will outlive even the earth itself.

One of the very great achievements of this century has been the discovery of the DNA molecules structured within the core of all living organisms. This source of all biological information, which forms the main constituent of our genes and chromosomes, is the universal code from which the enormous variety of life forms, from bacteria to man, have evolved. DNA's most extraordinary property is its capacity to adapt, regenerate, and self-perpetuate. Because of this capacity, the information contained in DNA is literally millions and millions of years old, yet shows no sign of aging.

The ability of living systems to maintain stability and continuity amidst great upheavals speaks for the intelligence that underlies and organizes their existence. If that intelligence is powerful enough to allow for the immortality of a species and immortality within certain single-cell organisms, such as bacteria (which divide continuously and thus never die), is it possible for immortality to be structured within an individual human being?

In an age in which great scientific discoveries are natural, even common, there are leading researchers in the field of aging who feel that extending longevity—even in the direction of immortality—is entirely possible. One of the world's top gerontologists, Dr. Bernard Strehler, wrote a prophetic essay early in his life:

> Immortality—that magic word is, I believe, the key to the direction which will be taken in the next great step forward in science. From time immemorial man has sought without avail a way to eliminate or reverse the effects of time on the human body. . . . I have come to one conclusion—that senility and death are not the inevitable ends of human existence, either as individuals or as a race, and that through scientific research we shall eventually be able to remove the sorrows of death from the human mind.

While there are a few gerontologists who find it difficult to understand why the body ages at all, most see aging as an inevitable part of life. Immortality to them is a just an imaginary idea, not a subject for serious study. However, the whole process of human development is an incredibly creative one. All our mental and physical functions are constantly improving to some optimal level until the age of twenty or thirty, and then it all changes. We begin to age. Why? The answer to this question is, of course, central to locating the nature of immortality. Let's first examine this question from the point of view of several different theories in modern physiology, which emphasize the physiology of matter, and then from the perspective of Maharishi's Vedic Physiology, which emphasizes the role of the physiology of consciousness.

Why Do We Age?

Two basic theories of aging are prevalent today: aging is due either to a predetermined genetic program or "clock," or to the accumulation of errors and the gradual breakdown of the system.

According to the genetic clock theory, the damage or disorders seen in older organisms are not the result of a random or accidental process, but rather of a specific genetic program. For example, Dr. Strehler believes that the process of aging is similar to other stages of development and is controlled by a specific set of "aging genes." When the aging genes are activated, they regulate the gradual breakdown of the organism. Just as other developmental stages are orchestrated by the information in DNA, so too is aging.

According to the error theory, aging occurs because the organism is unable to properly repair errors that accumulate over time. The precise cause of this accumulation of errors is a subject of great debate among researchers. As a result, error theory itself has led to many different theories of aging.

One theory of aging that seems to integrate many divergent viewpoints identifies free radicals, which we discussed in the previous chapter, as the cause of aging. Dr. Richard Cutler, working at Baltimore's prestigious Gerontology Research Center, part of the National Institute of Aging at NIH, is one of many scientists investigating free-radical reactions. In an interview several years ago in a popular magazine, Dr. Cutler maintained, "There's not one shred of evidence for any bottleneck on the evolution of human longevity. How can we keep building new and wonderful machines while we've stayed the same for a hundred thousand years? Our first priority must be to control man's aging process and from that all other things will flow."

Dr. Cutler and others believe that to increase longevity, all that is necessary is to alter a small number of genes so that the body is better able—through the increased production of antioxidants—to combat the metabolic damage caused by free radicals. One approach Dr. Cutler is investigating is to use pharmaceutical agents to stimulate the cells to produce more antioxidants. The effects of this approach on humans, however, are still unknown. When asked about his own life-extension program and whether or not he would consider injecting himself with one of the chemicals he now studies in animals, Dr. Cutler replied: "Not yet, I'm afraid of it. These substances could turn out to be dangerous."

While many life-extension scientists may express great optimism in some new drug or in genetic engineering, they also realize the potential danger of tampering with the body's inner ecology.

A Delicate Ecology

Perhaps the most important fact we have learned from modern research is that the body is a highly delicate ecology. When you introduce a new drug, each person reacts differently. In one individual, a certain dosage will produce no bad side effects. In another individual, it may come close to being lethal.

This is the same problem we have faced with the introduction of chemicals and pollutants into the environment. We just can't predict how the environment will react. There are so many interacting layers of animals and plants, so many internal systems of regulation and feedback, all striving to maintain balance. When DDT was first introduced, it was considered to be a miracle. It was, and still is, used extensively in many areas of the world, particularly to kill mosquitoes that spread malaria. For years, no one had any idea of the vast ecological consequences of this one chemical. When they did find out, the news was not encouraging. DDT doesn't just disappear with the mosquitoes. It stays around, penetrating more and more layers of world ecology and causing more and more havoc.

Precisely the same problem exists in medicine. Every new wonder drug creates initial hope and enthusiasm until time goes on and scientists reveal more and more adverse side effects. One of the most interesting cases is the drug cortisone. When this drug first appeared, it created great hope for curing disease and prolonging life. It was thought to be the wonder drug of the century, particularly for older people with inflammatory diseases. For example, in conditions such as arthritis, an injection of cortisone can have the very dramatic effect of reducing pain and inflammation. Unfortunately, a long list of negative side effects was later discovered, including possible death. The doctor thus faces a dilemma: the prolonged use of cortisone can greatly reduce pain and discomfort, and at the same time can cause such abnormalities as brittle bones, increased infections, marked distortions of the face and body, and other serious disorders.

In the *Physicians' Desk Reference*, a handbook for physicians, lists of the harmful side effects of drugs go on for literally thousands of pages. The body is not simply a collection of replaceable chemicals, but an extremely complex ecology, whose state of health and life span are directly related to how we treat it.

Balance: The Inner Wisdom of the Body

We have developed a very impatient and combative attitude in our problem-solving approach in the field of health and aging. Our sense of long-term planning, whether it applies to our own individual lives or to our overall environment, is very limited. We tend to favor immediate solutions: if you overeat and feel pain, take Alka-Seltzer; if you overwork and get a headache, take an aspirin; if you get too stressed and can't sleep, take Valium; if you want to live longer, take some new wonder drug.

It's a very strange philosophy of life—one which puts us always at odds with the natural tendencies of our physiology. We feel we can do whatever we want and then take a drug or have an operation to correct the consequences.

For example, we know that heart disease is preventable, but we continue to do the very things that aggravate the condition, almost as if we are challenging natural law. Technology is our savior; if our arteries become clogged, we can replace them with new ones. This same careless "godlike" attitude has also crept into the field of gerontology.

Gerontologists can be very bold, feeling that it's only a matter of time before they create a wonder drug that will defy death and ensure immortality.

When I listen to the claims of gerontologists seeking to unlock the gates of immortality, I am genuinely interested. Because of my own scientific training, I appreciate their logic, and I have no question about their sincerity or belief that life extension is possible, for I share this belief. But what I do object to is their purely mechanistic attitude and approach.

The body is a hierarchical network of interlocking feedback systems. The primary function of these systems is to maintain balance and internal stability. They resist every attempt to manipulate them by chemical means. If you increase someone's levels of a certain hormone by injecting it into him, his body's intricate feedback systems will resist the outside change—they will compensate by increasing or decreasing production of the hormone, to keep it at its predetermined set point. Of course, if the drug is powerful enough and taken in a sufficient dosage, it acts like an atomic bomb on the system. The body can't defend itself and is overwhelmed. Some of its reactions may be beneficial, especially in relieving acute symptoms. However, many of its other reactions may result in devastating side effects.

How, then, can top gerontologists believe that life extension is merely a matter of artificially increasing a hormone, taking some new wonder drug, or manipulating a few genes? With numerous theories about the aging process, each offering a new potion, it becomes quite difficult to know which program really does influence longevity.

In an article on life-extension programs published a few years ago in the *New England Journal of Medicine*, the author clearly points out that almost all the current so-called life-extension programs, while widely publicized, have not been shown to produce beneficial effects in humans. He goes on to warn of their potential side effects. It would be folly not to heed his caution: "Any attempts to intervene in aging processes in human beings must carefully weigh the risks of potential adverse responses."

In an age of genetic engineering there is an enormous potential for both oversight and undersight. As we gain deeper knowledge into the laws of nature and develop the technology to tamper with these laws, our responsibility for proper and holistic judgment increases beyond any expectation.

We must remember that the body possesses its own inner intelligence. For any effective longevity program to be safe and complete, it must use and enliven this inner wisdom of the body. Maharishi Ayur-Ved offers procedures to realign the individual physiology with the sequential unfoldment of the impulses of natural law that uphold the universe. The first statement in the Charak Samhita, a classic medical text of Ayur-Ved, reads:

Athato dirghan jivitiyam
adhyayam vyakhyasyamah

We shall now expound the chapter
on the "Quest for Longevity."

The Vedic texts also state: *Ayur-Ved amritanam*—"Ayur-Ved is for immortality." In order to prolong life, Maharishi Ayur-Ved prescribes many different techniques that influence both the physiology of matter and the physiology of consciousness.

In the last chapter we discussed the research on the numerous beneficial effects of the natural herbal preparation Maharishi Amrit Kalash on free radicals and the aging process. There have also been a number of studies on the effects of the consciousness approach of Maharishi Ayur-Ved, the TM and TM-Sidhi program, on aging and longevity.

The Effects of the Transcendental Meditation and TM-Sidhi Program on the Aging Process

Studies on aging conducted at Duke University have correlated seven factors with aspects of aging and longevity. These are, in order of significance: cardiovascular disease, work satisfaction, cigarette smoking, physical function, happiness rating, self-health rating, and performance IQ.

Studies on people who regularly practice the Transcendental Meditation technique show improvements in all seven factors. Cardiovascular disease risk factors such as high blood pressure and high cholesterol levels improve. Job satisfaction improves. Cigarette smoking and alcohol consumption decrease. Physical functions (such as motor reactions, respiratory and circulatory functions, and sensory performance) improve. Meditators show increased happiness ratings, contentment, self-regard, and self-actualization, and decreased anxiety and neuroticism. Increased happiness is further demonstrated by the significant improvement in hospitalized patients suffering from severe depression. (These findings are also of interest in light of a study conducted at Harvard University, which clearly establishes that better mental health is associated with longevity.) Meditators also show improvements in self-health ratings and on IQ tests designed to measure fluid intelligence.

Other studies have focused directly on measuring biological markers of the aging process in elderly TM subjects. What is biological aging and how is it different from chronological aging? The concept is very simple. We all know someone, perhaps a grandmother or aunt, who chronologically is over 60, but whose physical energy and mental alertness—her biological age—resembles that of a 40-year-old. She is spry, lively, and in excellent physical condition. On the other hand, there is the 40-year-old businessman who does not look "young" anymore. In fact his blood pressure and heart functioning suggest that he is closer to 60. We see it all the time. The fact is that different people age in different ways. Part of the reason is genetic, but most of it is how we live life.

The most common method of measuring biological age is a battery of physiological and psychological tests that measure such things as memory, blood pressure, hearing ability, and reaction time. These tests involve varying degrees of complexity, ease of administration, and utility of results.

One of the first studies on the effect of the Transcendental Meditation and TM-Sidhi program on biological aging used three of the most common aging measurements: near point vision, hearing at higher frequencies, and systolic blood pressure. The U.S. Public Health Service has gathered extensive data on aging using these measures; reliable normal values have been established for all age groups.

The study found that long-term TM meditators had significantly younger biological ages than short-term meditators, controls, and norms for the general population, and that the strength of this effect was related to the length of practice of the TM technique. Long-term practitioners of the TM and TM-Sidhi program had biological ages that were on average twelve years younger than their chronological ages. (The average chronological age was 54; the average biological age was 42.) Two studies conducted in England have replicated and extended these initial findings. In one cross-sectional study, TM subjects were found to have biological ages seven years younger on average than their chronological ages. A follow-up study 1.5 years later found that the biological ages of the same meditators had actually decreased by another 1.5 years.

Another important recent study on biological aging involved the measurement of one of the most reliable biochemical markers of the aging process, serum levels of the adrenal androgen, dehydroepiandrosterone sulfate (DHEA-S). DHEA-S rises throughout childhood and adolescence, attains peak levels during the mid-twenties, and then declines progressively with age. By the eighth and ninth decades of life, one's DHEA-S level may have declined by 80%.

DHEA-S levels were measured in 270 men and 153 women who were experienced participants in the Transcendental Meditation and TM-Sidhi program, and compared according to gender and five-year age groups to 799 men and 453 women who were not meditating. The mean DHEA-S levels in the meditators were significantly higher than in the controls, in all 11 of the age groups measured in women, and in 6 of 7 groups in men over 40. Statistical analysis using TM-group data revealed that this effect was independent of diet, body mass index, and exercise. The mean TM-group levels measured in all the women and in the older men were generally comparable to levels in control groups 5 to 10 years younger.

Studies have shown that low levels of DHEA-S are associated with cardiovascular disease, breast cancer, and obesity. That regular practitioners of Maharishi's Transcendental Meditation technique show higher DHEA-S levels than control populations is another indicator of better health and younger biological age in TM participants.

A well-controlled study conducted at Harvard University considered the effects of Transcendental Meditation on health, longevity, and cognitive and behavioral flexibility in elderly individuals. Seventy-three residents of homes for the elderly (60 women and 13 men, with a mean age of 80.7 years) were randomly assigned to a no-treatment group or to one of three programs: the TM program, mindfulness training (an active distinction-making procedure), and a relaxation program. These programs were designed to be equivalent in external structure and to foster similar expectation of results.

All groups had similar pretest measurements, yet after a three-month experimental period, the TM group had significantly improved in comparison with one or more of the other groups on three measures of cognitive flexibility: the Overlearned Verbal Task, the Stroop Color-Word Interference Test, and the Associate Learning Test. Improvements were seen in word fluency, systolic blood pressure (using two types of measurements), self-reported measures of aging and behavioral flexibility, and (after 18 months) in nurses' ratings of mental health. Also, TM subjects reported feeling more interested during their practice, and better and more relaxed immediately after their practice, than did the active-thinking and relaxation subjects. Overall, more TM subjects found their practice to be personally valuable than did members of the other treatment groups.

The most striking finding was that in addition to reversing age-related decline, TM appeared to directly enhance longevity: all members of the TM group were still alive three years after the program began, in contrast with an average 76.6% survival rate for the other groups and a 62.5% survival rate for residents in the same facilities who were not included in the study.

Finally, two recent studies have investigated the effects of the TM and TM-Sidhi program on neurophysiological activity in the elderly. The investigators used a sensory evoked potential measurement known as the P300 response, which occurs when the brain is attending to novel stimuli. The time it takes for the P300 to appear following a stimulus, known as the latency of the P300, increases with age. Both studies showed that elderly TM subjects exhibited shorter latency of the P300 response compared to controls, again demonstrating younger biological age.

The results of these studies on biological aging, supported by the large number of other physiological studies, strongly indicate that the Transcendental Meditation and TM-Sidhi program retards and even reverses the aging process.

Promoting Immortality in Change

Maharishi emphasizes that at its most profound level, the level of the unified field of natural law, the physiology of consciousness is immortal. It is in the mechanism of manifestation, the transformation from the physiology of consciousness to physiology of matter, that the seeds of aging are sowed. As we saw in the discussion of pragya-aparadh, the mistake of the intellect, in Chapter 6, some impurity or imbalance can occur when the unmanifest field of consciousness expresses itself into the basic tendencies or channels of life. Another example of this phenomenon in physiology is seen when even one or a few abnormalities in the sequence of nucleotides in DNA can result in fatal diseases—for example, sickle cell anemia. "Evolution," Maharishi comments, "is certainly a system of change, but the system of change does not have to be dragging to life, because the change also is structured in nonchange." Change in reality is only an excitation of the non-changing unified field. In the process of evolution, due to the mistake of the intellect, the field of nonchange appears as change—the unchanging nature of the unified field is hidden from view by all the changing diversity of creation. However, as Maharishi quotes from the Vedic literature, "The son of immortality does not have to be mortal." All that is necessary to reverse the mistake of the intellect is an unimpeded flow of intelligence throughout our physiology of consciousness and our physiology of matter.

This is the viewpoint of the Vedic paradigm. Ignorance—forgetting our ability to experience and be in tune with the immortal nature of our physiology of consciousness—is the reason for aging. Maharishi states, "Enlightenment is just a matter of awakening. . . . Nothing happens in the state of enlightenment other than [we gain] the awareness of unboundedness, the awareness of immortality." It is only a process of remembering our inner nature, of waking up to our full unbounded potential.

For every state of consciousness, there is a corresponding state in the physiology. If consciousness is established on the level of perfect balance, then the physiology will reflect that quality. The orderly sequential flow of awareness will be accompanied by a corresponding orderly flow of physiological functioning. If there is some disruption or imbalance in the expression of the dynamics of consciousness, then that becomes manifest on the gross level of the physiology in the process of aging.

Maharishi explains that "when the awareness has no memory of the unbounded, then this is the aging process." He connects the process of aging with the inability to live in harmony with all the laws of nature: "Aging is directly associated with natural law, and if there is a violation of even a few of the laws of nature, then aging will keep on breathing." The prescription for immortality, then, is that "the totality of natural law has to become a living reality. When no aspect of natural law is violated, then immortality will be a continuum." Finally, Maharishi again strongly emphasizes that "lack of ability to incorporate the totality of natural law in every phase of living is the basic cause of aging." The result of violation of natural law is stress; we age as a result of the accumulation of stress, which prevents us from having access to the total potential of natural law in higher states of consciousness.

In higher states of consciousness, the underlying unity of life, the unified field of all natural law, is the permanent reality of our lives. The sequential unfoldment of the laws of nature is perfectly orderly and balanced in this state. All the procedures of Maharishi Ayur-Ved, especially the Transcendental Meditation and TM-Sidhi program, are designed to enable each individual to naturally and effortlessly achieve higher states, live in tune with the total potential of natural law, and therefore not violate any laws of nature. Thus in the Vedic paradigm, the simplest and most practical formula for disallowing aging is to become enlightened.

PART 3

THE PHYSIOLOGY
OF SOCIETY

THE WEEK WAR ENDED

H IS EXCELLENCY WILL SEE YOU NOW."

The voice startled me, so intent was I on trying to hear any sound from the outside world. Even artillery fire would be muffled where we were, I decided. This was my first visit to a dictator's bunker. Looking around when we first arrived, I was surprised to find it decorated with comfortable overstuffed chairs and plush carpeting. One hardly noticed that the curtains had no windows behind them, not even slits.

"If you'll step this way," the guard murmured. I trailed behind the small group that rose to follow him. We were a delegation of three American scientists visiting Central America on a peace mission. We had come to Nicaragua in response to a plea that had appeared in the press from the citizens of a town devastated by the violence of a brutal civil war. The people were calling for any national or international agency to bring relief: "Anyone who can help, please help." Maharishi wanted to respond immediately. We arrived in this small nation more or less unannounced, but after several phone calls were granted an audience with its head of state.

Peace was a good calling-card just then. After years of using the country as his own private reserve, El Presidente's rule was rapidly crumbling. The rebel forces, labeled as Communists by the government and as liberators by themselves, were gathering outside the capital. The final assault was expected at any time. Many thought it was overdue.

When we entered a large office, the face that greeted us was instantly recognizable from the six o'clock news back home as the country's president.

"If you don't mind," the president gestured toward chairs near his desk. Then he returned to the phone conversation we had interrupted. He was a large, imposing man, impeccably dressed in a three-piece silk suit.

"Don't worry, Tom," he said into the phone, "the situation is completely under control. There's a little trouble, it's nothing we can't handle. We are still very interested in making the deal." I gathered that he was talking, not to a field commander, but to an old friend in the United States. Years ago the president had made connections at Harvard Business School. Now he apparently assumed that he could still run his country on the basis of business as usual.

I marveled at the unreality of his view. In October 1978, the decay of power was in the very air of Nicaragua. The day before, we had visited its parliamentary chambers. Terrorists had recently sprayed the building with machine-gun fire. I looked up and noticed hundreds of bullet holes in the elaborately decorated ceiling. On the way to the bunker, we had seen armed soldiers in combat fatigues on every corner.

When his phone call was over, the president asked us to begin. There was a brief pause. None of us had ever been in quite this position before. The first to speak was Dr. Lawrence Domash, a Princeton-trained physicist who headed our group. "We are American scientists who have come to brief you," he began, "on a new technology that can bring peace to your country."

The dictator nodded. He did not seem perturbed, or for that matter surprised.

"We are a special group formed to bring about world peace," Dr. Domash said. "Approximately 150 of this group are living in the hotel there"—he gestured in the direction where a window would have faced our hotel, if a window had been there—"and at this moment we are using this new technology to calm hostilities within your nation."

"What exactly are you doing?" the man asked.

"We are meditating. That is the core of this technology. It is the first technology of its kind, based entirely upon consciousness. But I would like to lay out our proposal for you in full. May I?" He began to bring out some papers.

"Please," the president said politely.

We brought out a copy of that week's local newspaper and held it up for him to see. On the front page was a picture of a large group of young men, most of them under thirty, all dressed in coats and ties, all smiling.

"As you can see from the coverage," Dr. Domash pointed to the story, "we announced our intention on the day of our arrival to prove that we could bring peace to your nation." He handed over more recent issues of the same paper. "Our formal research results will not be forthcoming for several months, but as you can see from these accounts, your press has in fact reported a drop-off in war-related incidents since our arrival. This is an article commenting on the sudden lull in hostilities that has begun."

I wondered if "war" was the word the president would have chosen to describe current events, but it passed without comment.

"Because this technology cools down negative tendencies of all kinds," Dr. Domash continued, "we also expect from our past experience that you will see a decrease in crime, particularly here in the capital, and extending to other parts of the country. Also, hospital admissions and road accidents should have decreased in the past week. Relations with neighboring countries could suddenly improve. All of these benefits will continue, we feel certain, so long as the meditators maintain their presence here."

The man leafed through the papers, then silently handed them back.

"Presently," Dr. Domash said, "similar lulls in hostility and even cease-fires are being created in southern Africa, the Middle East, and Southeast Asia. Sometime during this month or next, in order to demonstrate conclusively that this technology works, we hope to see a halt in all major conflicts around the world."

Since the dictator continued to regard us with polite interest, we began to relax. Two days before, we had boarded a jet in Miami, scheduled to stop in several Central and South American countries. Many of them were military "hot spots." The meditators involved in our peace efforts had preceded us into the region by about two weeks. The majority were based nearby, but smaller groups had quietly taken positions in the neighboring countries.

Because we felt convinced that we were on the verge of changing mankind's whole concept of political power, everyone was committed to bringing our project to the attention of national leaders, no matter what their reactions might be. We felt confident in the influence we could create, even though we had never before confronted a ruling head of state with our aims.

The Meissner Effect

Dr. Domash continued, "Essentially we are taking advantage of well-known principles that apply in physics. But we are applying them to a new area. In physics, Newton's third law of thermodynamics holds that if you decrease the temperature of a physical system, then the system increases in orderliness. Ice, for example, is a more orderly and stable form of H_2O than water.

"Moreover, if you have an impurity dissolved in the water, such as salt, the water will spontaneously purify itself as it freezes. In a glass of salt water, as the temperature is lowered towards the freezing point, a layer of salt is deposited in the bottom, and you are left with a mass of ice above it that is pure H_2O.

"A group of meditators can produce orderliness the same way. Violence, hostility, and the collapse of law and order are disorderly expressions of consciousness in a society. If you can cool down the collective level of awareness, then collective consciousness can restore itself to orderliness, just as the water can rid itself of the salt and form a stable, orderly structure of ice crystals."

I watched the dictator carefully while Dr. Domash talked. It was obvious that he caught on, at least partially, to what was being presented. This in itself was an achievement. We knew that from the viewpoint of conventional politics, we had come from the moon. We wanted to convey that what we actually represented was an entirely new perspective.

The future of the nation did not lie with El Presidente or with the rebels. Each looked upon the other as an implacable enemy, but in fact they had one common enemy—their own chaotic consciousness.

Dr. Domash went on, "A more profound example of the principle of reducing activity and thus increasing orderliness and purity is seen in the phenomena of superfluidity and superconductivity. If the temperature of liquid helium is decreased to a few degrees above absolute zero, an extraordinary phase transition occurs, producing a unique fourth state of matter different from the gaseous, liquid, or solid states—known as the superfluid state. In this superfluid state, helium can escape through glass containers; it becomes as if unbounded. Its resistance to flow is zero, and its capacity to conduct heat is infinite.

"If the temperature of a metal, such as lead, is reduced to a few degrees above absolute zero, a similar type of phase transition occurs, resulting in the phenomenon of superconductivity. One of the unique properties of a superconductor is its property of invincibility, known as the Meissner Effect. When a magnetic field is brought near an ordinary conductor of electricity, it penetrates into the interior of the conductor and disturbs the flow of electrons inside. On the other hand, when a magnetic field is brought near a superconductor, the superconductor produces a magnetic field that precisely cancels the intruding field. The result is that no external magnetic field can penetrate into the superconductive region. This same principle applies to a nation. By utilizing the Transcendental Meditation and TM-Sidhi program, we can create a highly coherent state in the collective consciousness such that no damaging outside force can penetrate."

In our delegation was Dr. David Orme-Johnson, one of the first researchers to study the collective effects of the Transcendental Meditation and TM-Sidhi program. He was the next to talk to the president. Dr. Orme-Johnson opened up a map of Central America with certain regions marked in red. "As you can see, we have placed a core group of meditators here to create the desired cooling effect on hostilities. Smaller groups have been positioned in neighboring countries. They are not large enough to create an effect on their own, but they strengthen it from the outside.

"We are proposing to leave these groups in place for the next two months," Dr. Orme-Johnson explained, "so that the government will have time, if it is satisfied with the results, to assume responsibility for continuing the project.

"In each country we need to train meditators, enough so that the effect will persist. In the beginning, that would amount to instructing a large number of people, up to one percent of the population. We would supply the teachers; all we ask is that you reimburse us for our expenses.

"However, the numbers can be drastically reduced. The meditators are now practicing a much more powerful technique called the TM-Sidhi program. We could begin to teach this technique within the next year, and then only a core group, of less than three hundred people, could maintain peace in your country."

This would be the stickiest point, we knew. Although he looked very tired and under tremendous strain, the dictator had listened to us. Now we expected him to act. It often happened, when we presented our program, that government officials showed tremendous enthusiasm while we were physically with them. We expected to hear from them afterwards, but there would be only silence. The gap between their situation and the solution we were presenting was too great for them to bridge alone.

Transcendental Meditation is regarded as a means for self-development. From the start, however, Maharishi taught that it had much wider implications. At a time when Westerners were just absorbing the idea that their own consciousness could be developed individually, Maharishi posed an incisive analysis of unrest on the social scale:

"Where there is disagreement and dissension in families or in a group of friends, the disharmony seems to occur only in a small area. Individuals do not realize that through ill-feeling, malice, bad behavior, harsh words, and suffering, they are contributing to the disruption and destruction of the peace of the world."

The Vedic paradigm places the individual at the center of the world, proposing that the unit of world unrest is each individual; therefore, the unit of world peace must also be the same:

"The problem of world peace can be solved," Maharishi explains, "only by solving the problem of the individual's peace, and the problem of the individual's peace can only be solved by creating in him a state of happiness."

Maharishi presented this simple logic in 1963 in his first book, *Science of Being and Art of Living*. He had been stating it to audiences from the first day when he walked out from the Himalayas and began to teach TM. Whatever the public thought he was accomplishing, Maharishi measured his success by one standard—bringing peace to every single person in the world. In the early years, his strategy had been utterly direct: he intended to teach Transcendental Meditation to as many people as possible in every country on earth. By raising their standard of happiness, he would raise the happiness of mankind. It was a strategy of pure numbers.

By the early 1970s, however, his strategy had become much broader. He had successfully "multiplied" himself, as he liked to put it, by training a large, dedicated corps of Transcendental Meditation teachers. But even with many teachers, it was obvious that getting the whole world to meditate would take too long. Even though he saw the decrease of stress and negativity in the consciousness of meditators, there was obviously growing tension in the world as a whole.

The Maharishi Effect

The progress toward world peace needed to take a quantum leap, and in 1974 it did just that. By that time, Transcendental Meditation was being practiced on a wide enough scale that some cities in the United States had one percent or more of their populations meditating. Examining the statistics from four Midwestern college towns, the original "one percent cities," psychologist Garland Landrith observed a decrease of crime in those areas once they reached the one percent threshold.

This was an intriguing finding, since crime was on the upsurge nationally and had in fact become a major domestic issue. The Upanishads and other Vedic texts that describe the practice of meditation declare that yogis or swamis produce calming influences on their surroundings. Maharishi had suggested as early as 1961 that TM would be found to have this effect.

Landrith's observation prompted a formal study, begun by him and colleague Candace Borland in December 1974. They took all the one percent cities existing in the U.S. in 1972, a total of 11, and analyzed their crime rates in comparison with control cities. Like the one percent cities, the controls were college towns with populations between 25,000 and 50,000, located in various parts of the country. The matching was done precisely according to population demographics. The researchers wanted to isolate the TM variable as accurately as possible.

They discovered that during the years 1972–73, the FBI reported an average decrease in crime of 8.2% in the cities with 1% meditators, compared with an actual increase of 8.3% for the control cities. Overall, this represented a difference of 16.5%. The researchers also noted that the chance of this being a random occurrence, a fluke, was only one in 1,000. The conclusion was that TM could reduce negative tendencies in the environment, and that the threshold of the effect seemed to be one percent—that was the percentage of meditators required for the effect to work. The scientists appropriately named this phenomenon "the Maharishi Effect." A later analysis confirmed that a sudden drop in crime rate occurred as soon as any city crossed the one percent mark. The decrease held firm, on average, for at least six years.

Scientists theorized that some type of phase transition must be occurring in the general awareness of society. As soon as a core number of meditators created orderliness in the collective consciousness of society, orderliness increased everywhere. The decrease in crime was really just a ripple on the surface. The real action took place at a subtler level.

Maharishi called the subtler level "collective consciousness," the sum of the consciousnesses of all the people in the society. In the past, collective consciousness has never been studied in a serious scientific manner, because it could be neither isolated nor experimentally experienced. The most sophisticated sociological theories give at best a vague description of a social field as an interlocking network of social and behavioral interactions within specific economic and environmental conditions.

The Vedic paradigm removes misconceptions and ambiguities, presenting the concept of collective consciousness from a more complete perspective. We have not only an individual physiology, but a collective physiology—the physiology of society—in which each of us is like one cell in a large superorganism. The physiology of society has its own physiology of consciousness and its own physiology of matter. Its physiology of consciousness encompasses the collective consciousness of all the individuals. Its physiology of matter encompasses all material activities of all individuals.

In the case of the one percent studies, the physiology of society under consideration was that of a community or city. But the effect did not have a theoretical limit. If it could influence positive trends in society, then it might also be applicable to a nation or even the world. On the world scale, the equivalent of crime is terrorism and war. Therefore, if the meditators exerted a coherent enough influence, they should accomplish something amazing—they should put an end to war.

The Extended Maharishi Effect

When he introduced it in 1976, Maharishi explained that his TM-Sidhi program, particularly the TM-Sidhi technique of Yogic Flying (described in Chapter 10), was an even more powerful technology for enlivening the unified field of natural law than Transcendental Meditation. He predicted that on this basis, a comparatively small number of people—the square root of one percent of a population—practicing this program in groups should be sufficient to produce measurable effects on the various quality-of-life indices in any society.

The rationale for this prediction came from discussions with leading physicists concerning coherent effects seen in physical systems, particularly in the laser. Normal light is emitted in direct proportion to the number of atoms in the light source. Each atom emits a photon when it is excited and then returns to its ground state. When the atoms in a laser are in perfect correlation with each other, then a new type of collective behavior, characterized by macroscopic orderliness, emerges. The atoms cease to act independently and instead behave as one complete, coherent system. As a result, the intensity of the light emitted by the laser of N atoms is magnified enormously, to N squared (N^2). Thus, if 100 atoms are perfectly in phase with one another in the laser, they will radiate with an intensity of 100^2, or 10,000 times that of a single atom. This phenomenon is known in physics as superradiance.

This was the effect we were testing during this world peace project in many parts of the world. In most places we did not have enough TM-Sidhi experts to create a total cessation of war. We were closest to the square root of one percent in Lebanon and Nicaragua, and there the hostilities suddenly dropped off—some observers said it was as if a switch had been pulled. This was the first large-scale experiment testing the "square root of one percent" effect, which became known as the Extended Maharishi Effect.

The purpose of our presentation to the Central American dictator, however, was not to propose a scientific experiment, but to offer to stop war in his country and create a thriving and peaceful society. Unfortunately, it was clear that we were not getting through. The huge gulf between the dictator's world and the one we were sketching was obvious to all of us in the room. At a certain point, after we had been talking for perhaps an hour, a phone call came, and he excused himself to take it.

I leaned over to Dr. Orme-Johnson. "What can we do?" I whispered. "I think we're losing him."

"Do anything," he said. "Give him your slide show."

Indeed that was about all the ammunition we had left. When the president turned to face us, I introduced myself as a physiologist.

"I realize," I began, "that what we've told you seems very abstract." The expression on his face indicated how right I was.

"There is another side to meditation that is not abstract at all," I said as I set up the projector. "I have been conducting research on TM and stress. What I have found will interest you."

Lights dimmed. I flashed a slide on the wall that illustrated the decline of blood lactate during Transcendental Meditation. The next slide showed EEG measurements, emphasizing the alpha-wave peaks of meditators. To me, these are rather technical, but for the first time the man looked fascinated.

"Show me more of that, if you would."

There was a lot more to show—all of the many findings on Transcendental Meditation. I explained the EEG changes in detail because these results establish the high degree of coherence that is established within the individual.

As slides of more and more findings appeared on the wall, I made the point that these were the first modern proofs that the age-old practice of meditation had scientific validity. I pointed out, as tactfully as possible, that if Americans could benefit from reduced stress through meditation, then certainly his own people could.

"Stress is within the individual," I said, "but it is also out there in the environment. War and civil unrest are expressions of collective stress, and what we are offering is a way to reduce it."

"Yes, yes," he responded eagerly.

"If one person can use this meditation to reach a level of consciousness where he does not suffer from stress, then could an entire nation not benefit even more?"

It was the closest we dared come to saying, "Look, you and this country are in deep trouble. Let us help."

The man sat thoughtfully. Then he stood and congratulated us on our presentation. He seemed genuinely impressed and completely persuaded. He warmly shook my hand as we left, promising that he would be in touch soon. It even occurred to me that he might become the first government leader in history to support a nationwide program to create coherence in collective consciousness. We waited for his call, and then, because of the high cost of maintaining many groups of TM-Sidhi experts in these trouble spots all over the world, the group had to leave. It was not entirely surprising to hear that within months he had been violently deposed and rebel leaders were now firmly in power.

The World Peace Project

Flying over the aqua waters of the Caribbean on the way to Central America, we had considered the risks we were running. Maharishi's TM-Sidhi experts were deliberately stepping into places that could erupt into full-scale violence at any time. Some of the hot spots in the world that year included Iran, Lebanon, Nicaragua, and Southern Rhodesia (now Zimbabwe).

Every location was crackling with tension, especially in Iran. At one point, the hotel in Tehran where the meditators were based appeared to be under siege. Mobs opposed to the Shah were pillaging the city, concentrating on the sections where foreigners resided.

The job of the scientists was to explain the principles of the Extended Maharishi Effect to the heads of state in each country. Transcendental Meditation had undergone scientific scrutiny for more than a decade. By the time our delegation met with the various government leaders, there was a core of research findings that strongly validated our claims about the scientific mechanisms involved in creating world peace.

The research also gave us credentials in the countries we visited and helped explain the otherwise baffling phenomenon that one observer called "an outbreak of peace." Looking back now, I cannot help but admire the meditators' commitment and dedication to creating world peace. I later read in the newspaper a first-hand account of the Iran peace project by Jon Levy of Ithaca, New York:

> The forty of us were volunteers—freedom fighters, if you will—only the freedom we were fighting for was the freedom to be happy and to live without fear, and the fighting was done in a seated position with eyes closed. Teachers of the Transcendental Meditation program experienced in the TM-Sidhi program were being sent to Iran by His Holiness Maharishi Mahesh Yogi, the founder of the TM program, to change the chaos to harmony and the disorder to orderliness. . . .
>
> Seeing the degree of chaos that prevailed made the task seem almost impossible. True, I had seen a profound transformation in my own life and in others I instructed in the TM technique. And I had seen studies which show the environmental value of a small percentage of people gaining that level of "least excitation of consciousness" through the TM program: reduced crime rates, lower admissions to hospitals, less violence, and increased quality of life.
>
> But this was something else. This was tanks and machine guns on one side and fanaticism and Molotov cocktails on the other. When we arrived in Isfahan (a smaller city about 200 miles south of Tehran) . . . , we were welcomed by the sound of the hotel closest to ours being blown up and twelve of the city's banks being set aflame.
>
> And so there remained nothing to do but to get on with it. Tanks rumbled by our hotel as we settled into meditation and the TM-Sidhi program (an advanced series of techniques designed to develop perfect coordination between mind and body). As the first day turned into night, we began to sense a growing feeling of separateness from the turbulence going on around us. By the second day we were feeling very at ease, despite our external environment, and by the third day there was no denying the profound experience of "invincibility" which permeated everyone on the project. There was no fear, no anxiety, only a strong undercurrent of silence and peace.
>
> On the fourth day the value we had been experiencing overflowed into our environment. It could be easily noticed, even by those not in any way connected with our project. The sun came out, children returned to their play in the streets, the troops were not so much in evidence, the shops reopened, the cacophony of human and vehicular sounds which enunciate a healthy marketplace was, for the first time since we arrived, heard throughout the city. . . .
>
> Peace prevailed throughout the land. Nobody knew why. Almost nobody, anyway. As our inner experiences became even more pro-

found, the orderliness around us reflected that value. The tanks disappeared. The bazaars reopened. Schools throughout the country, which had been closed by the violence, again echoed with the cheerful voices of Iranian children. . . .

Perhaps the strongest single bit of evidence of our success occurred on "Army Day," an event which honors the national militia with parades and display of military hardware. It was thought opponents of . . . the Shah would seize the opportunity with a bloody confrontation. Instead, the people threw flowers at the passing troops, and no shots were fired anywhere in Iran that day.

Peace could be felt in every country the meditators visited. In Rhodesia, the rate of war deaths fell from an average of 16 per day to 3, starting the week the meditators arrived. In the countryside, 2,000 insurrectionists changed sides and enabled the transitional government to hold peaceful elections. Black leader Bishop Abel Muzorewa, flanked by guerrillas who had turned in their weapons, told an assembly, "Peace has at last taken hold of our war-torn society." The BBC's Iranian correspondent reported an inexplicable calm in the atmosphere after months of extreme chaos.

By the last weeks of December 1978, the World Peace Project was over. After maintaining some 1,400 meditators in hotels for an extended period, sometimes as long as four months, in groups ranging from 30 to 400 strong, financing had become an issue. We could not carry the burden of continuing the project without assistance. The various groups in Iran, Rhodesia, Nicaragua, and other countries were forced to pull out. There was some concern that if our influence made the cessation of hostilities possible, then our departure might easily tip the balance back the other way.

This appeared to happen in several places. War deaths in Rhodesia sprang from 3 per day back up to 16, the old level, as soon as the meditators left. A truce had begun in Lebanon in October, just as the meditation group responsible for that area landed in Israel. The truce lasted three months, making it one of the longest of the bloody civil war. When the group in Israel broke up in January, the truce collapsed, and war casualties immediately went up to pre-October levels.

In Iran the situation was potentially so explosive that removing the meditators at the end of four months had to be orchestrated like a military withdrawal. Maharishi told us that the peacemaking effect would collapse almost immediately after our groups left the country. Therefore, it was imperative to take them all home on the same day. Otherwise, an upsurge of violence could engulf any small group left behind.

We had groups scattered around the country, in Tehran, Isfahan, Tabriz, and Shiraz. To move them all out on the same day required that the groups in the south fly across the Persian Gulf at the same time that the northern and central groups flew to the Tehran airport. Then both contingents departed simultaneously for America on synchronized flights from Tehran and Saudi Arabia. Maharishi was emphatic about this maneuver, and we quickly understood why. Four days after our evacuation, mobs forced the Shah to flee Iran, and a few days later, amidst near chaos, the Ayatollah Khomeini returned from exile to assume power.

It is important to make it clear that we did not choose sides in any country we visited. Our personal opinions of the politics of the Shah or the Central American dictator (or the opinion of them held by the press) were not at issue. In all the volatile regions of the world, regimes rise and fall; ideologies follow each other in quick succession. Our concern was to create coherence in the collective consciousness. Maharishi explains that any government is only an "innocent mirror" of the collective consciousness of the people it governs. If collective consciousness is stressed and turbulent, the actions of the government will reflect that. In the current situation, creating coherence in collective consciousness through the Extended Maharishi Effect could not only end violence and suffering as quickly as possible, but it would transform any government, whatever its ideology, to be just and good.

The international news at the end of our project spoke to us in a way that no one else in the world could understand. On November 18, the *International Herald Tribune* quoted President Carter on his opinions about U.S.-Soviet relations: "I think that in recent weeks there has been an alleviation of tension between us, and I would like to see it continue." The president also commented that he did not know any concrete reason for the improvement.

Amid such scattered reports, including peace initiatives from the Soviet Union and the ratification of a historic treaty between China and Japan, a small item was carried in several American papers on November 30:

Despite border clashes, cold wars, internal turmoil, and lagging peace treaty negotiations, no nations are actively engaged in open warfare at the moment—a historic rarity.

That was the week war ended. This item was not data that scientists could use, but we remember it anyway.

There was, however, ample statistical data on the effects of the World Peace Project. One independent confirmation of the positive results came from evidence provided by the Conflict and Peace Data Bank (COPDAB), the largest data bank on international conflict and resolutions. This data, collected for over thirty years at the Center for International Development at the University of Maryland, was analyzed using a procedure known as content analysis. Two independent raters categorized news stories from a wide range of publications into areas such as hostile acts or cooperative events, based on a predetermined scale.

The COPDAB file showed that when the ten weeks during the World Peace Project were compared with the ten weeks before the project, there was a significant decrease in hostile acts in the trouble-spot areas (from 46.6% of all reported events to 29.5%), and a significant increase in cooperative acts (from 36% to 49.2%). When the ten-week period of the World Peace Project was compared with the same calendar period of the previous ten years (1968–77), it was again shown to be markedly more peaceful.

Obviously, the effect of peace was not permanent. The national governments we contacted did not choose to back the project with their own funds, although many officials had enthusiastically responded in private. A few of them even started TM. The scientists' data had confirmed that during the period of Maharishi's World Peace Project, a statistically significant reduction in hostility had taken place around the world—one which could not be accounted for either by chance or by previous political trends. The data confirmed that the technologies of the Vedic paradigm applied not only to the physiology of consciousness and the physiology of matter, but also to the physiology of society. They created coherence in the collective consciousness of society as a whole. These new technologies had demonstrated the power of consciousness to create world peace.

CHAPTER 10

THE NEUROPHYSIOLOGY
OF WORLD PEACE

P EOPLE CROWDED INTO THE MEETING ROOM AT THE
Washington Convention Center in Washington, D.C., on a
July morning in 1986, at what some observers called the
largest nonpolitical news conference in the city's history. Dr.
Bevan Morris, President of Maharishi International University, stood
at the podium; distinguished scientists were seated at a long table
beside him. More than 120 journalists and several TV crews were
there, representing every major North American television and radio
network, all the wire services, and most of the biggest newspapers and
magazines. All were awaiting an explanation—and an unprecedented
demonstration—of TM-Sidhi "Yogic Flying" and its role in creating
world peace.

"Today is the inauguration," began Dr. Morris, "of a program to
create world peace through a technology which creates coherence in
collective consciousness and neutralizes the stress in society."

"From Maharishi's perspective," he said, "we never wanted to display Yogic Flying." But the state of the world in the mid-1980s presented compelling reasons to do so: "With the rise of terrorism in the
world and the dangerous rivalry of the superpowers, Maharishi and all
of us feel a very urgent and pressing need to apply this technology to

166

create world peace for the sake of all mankind."

It is fascinating to recollect this discussion now. The context in which it was taking place was so vastly different from the one we know today. Only a few years ago the rivalry between the superpowers was a matter of the gravest concern. In Chapter 11 we'll explore the enormous changes in the world since 1986 in the context of the very program—Maharishi's Program to Create World Peace—presented at this historic press conference.

"No solution has ever been found to the problem of world peace," Dr. Morris continued. Treaties, international organizations, disarmament conferences, use of arms—nothing has ever worked. "Even as we speak," he said, "wars rage in the world. The world is covered by a pall of fear of war and terrorism and of the consequences in this nuclear age of the rivalry between the superpowers." What would be presented that day was the evidence of a practical program to fulfill the need for world peace—group practice of Maharishi's Transcendental Meditation and TM-Sidhi program, especially Yogic Flying.

Dr. Morris outlined the logic behind the principle that TM-Sidhi Yogic Flying can create world peace, first explaining Maharishi's viewpoint that war is caused by the build-up of stress in the collective consciousness of nations. "Every day in every nation, people are violating the laws of nature. . . . they are performing actions which injure themselves, their neighbors, and their environment. These wrong actions cause stress in the individual and society as a whole. . . . Stress in society can build up only to a certain point before the society explodes into some kind of calamity."

He referred to the research showing that Transcendental Meditation relieves stress in the individual, producing a more coherent, orderly, and efficient style of nervous system functioning. "What we are adding to this today," he said, "is the knowledge that practice of Maharishi's program by many people together in the same place, at the same time, relieves not only the individual's stresses but can relieve the stress in society as a whole." This, he pointed out, is especially the case with the advanced program of Transcendental Meditation, Maharishi's TM-Sidhi program, and he then explained some of the mechanics behind this effect.

"The TM-Sidhi techniques enhance the effect of Transcendental

Meditation in improving the coordination between mind and body. When these more powerful techniques are practiced by people together in groups, a coherent and orderly collective consciousness is created in society. The stress and incoherence in the life of the nation, which is the basic cause of world war, is eliminated."

The Yogic Flying technique is the most powerful of all the TM-Sidhi techniques, Dr. Morris said, again referring to research: "At the moment when the body is about to lift up during Yogic Flying, optimal coherence of brain functioning occurs." He also noted the research on the Maharishi Effect showing that coherence is produced throughout society by group practice of the technique by the square root of one percent of the population—even, as we saw in the previous chapter, "in the midst of war-torn environments where nothing else has worked." Finally, he described the broadest application of Maharishi's Program to Create World Peace—when 7,000 people (the square root of one percent of the world's population) practice the TM-Sidhi program together, they create the *global* Maharishi Effect, producing a peaceful influence throughout the whole of world consciousness.

Other speakers elaborated on the scientific research on the TM and TM-Sidhi program, Yogic Flying, and the Maharishi Effect. The audience was alert and attentive despite a veneer of understandable professional skepticism. Their wariness did not deter any of the speakers, including Dr. John Hagelin, who expounded brilliantly on the physics of Yogic Flying. Only from the level of the unified field of natural law, he said, could the phenomenon of Yogic Flying take place and the Maharishi Effect be produced.

Looking out at the assembled members of the press, I was encouraged by their response. They asked many questions of Dr. Hagelin and the others. They wanted to know all about Yogic Flying, the research on the Maharishi Effect, and, more importantly, they wanted to know how it could produce world peace.

After some time, everyone walked upstairs to the largest hall at the Convention Center for the Yogic Flying demonstration. Dr. Morris explained that it would be given at the finals of the North American Yogic Flying Competition in four events, complete with judges and timekeepers: the Yogic 25-meter hurdles, the Yogic 50-meter race, and the Yogic long and high jumps—all in the sitting position.

He also explained that, according to the classical texts of Vedic literature, Yogic Flying proceeds in three stages: "In the first, the body hops up into the air. The second stage is hovering, and the third stage is sustained flight." Twenty-two competitors from seven countries were participating; today they would be demonstrating the first, or hopping stage.

Twenty-five television camera crews and scores of photographers crowded the edges of the track—an acre of polyurethane foam covered in white sheets and divided by long red ribbons into five lanes. Again, I was surprised by the journalists' keen interest and seriousness as they covered what must have been one of the most unusual events of their careers.

Even with their enthusiasm, however, I must admit I was unsure of how it would come out on the six o'clock news. There was no telling what their senior editors, who had not been to the press conference, would do with the reports. This was just the kind of material that could easily be distorted in the media. I sat in front of the television that evening in eager anticipation: How much of the scientific research would they mention? Would they make fun of it all?

When the first reports appeared, I was deeply impressed. In fact, I was overjoyed. Every commentary was remarkably positive. It was a miracle. Here was a controversial topic that was being treated both objectively and comprehensively. More than 60 media organizations reported the news; their accounts of the Yogic Flying demonstration were printed in hundreds of publications and broadcast on scores of radio and television stations.

The Washington *Times* explained, "Theoretically, a yogic flyer has very orderly brain waves, fluid coordination between mind and body. Consciousness and matter become completely integrated, and all the coherence can spread around the world if enough meditators gather at the same time and place."

Some of the reporters shared their own enthusiasm for the significance of this historic event. I was especially struck by the remarks of Alex Van Oss on National Public Radio's "All Things Considered."

I've always wanted to fly, on my own, without tickets or seat belts.
And in my dreams as a child I did fly. I would climb a tree, jump, and
float back to ground, and sometimes with the right uplift to the chin, I

would even rise up over the trees at the end of the yard and the fields beyond and on up into the hills far away.

One Christmas, I asked for a real Superman suit, and it came with a note attached saying that of course, only the real Superman suit with its red cape could make you fly.

Dream on, Alex. And I have, these three decades. And I thought my dreams might come true this week when I got a leaflet from the World Assembly on Perfect Health, meeting at the Washington, D.C., Convention Center. It invited members of the media to a demonstration of what they called "Yogic Flying." There was a photo of two smiling young men in white shirts, practitioners of Maharishi Mahesh Yogi's Transcendental Meditation.

They were sitting cross-legged in the photo, sitting in lotus position and a good foot and a half off the ground. Superman, move over!

A couple of thousand spectators sat in the bleachers in the convention hall, and there were visiting dignitaries in turbans. There were dozens of photographers and camera technicians. And in one corner, a couple of meditators, with wires attached to their heads, surrounded by video monitors and people in white lab coats. The floor of the hall was a field of polyethylene foam pads covered with sheets and marked off in lanes just like an indoor race track.

At a press conference, spokesmen displayed graphs and gave out lists of scientific research papers saying that Transcendental Meditation, TM, when performed by enough people, had been shown to reduce the crime rate in a community, the number of auto accidents, suicides, and even raise stock prices.

Meanwhile, Bevan Morris, President of Maharishi International University in Iowa, said that through TM, when the brain waves are most coherent, the body can lift off the ground. The point of TM and Yogic Flying is to promote greater brain wave coherence and hence coherence in world consciousness, the basis of world peace. Governments have failed to do this, he said, the world is a mess; and that made it necessary to have this public demonstration, at least of the first stage of Yogic Flying. . . .

To be sure no one at the convention got beyond the hopping phase of Yogic Flying or even knew of anyone at stage two of levitation or three—free movements through the air. But it doesn't matter, they say. The techniques are thousands of years old, and there have been many masters in that time, surely. . . . I came away satisfied with a thought that when thousands of people gather, if only to meditate, if only to hop together, how could this not help but improve humanity's collective disposition. As for flying itself, it is a fact that in a certain field in Maryland thirty years ago, there was a boy who dreamed of flying through the rows of corn. He wore a Superman suit, with a red cape, and he was happy.

Quantum Effects in Consciousness and the Brain

The response of the media to Yogic Flying and to the explanation of the Global Maharishi Effect indicates the growing readiness and desire of people everywhere to gain a deeper understanding of the potential of consciousness. As we will see a little further on, the research on the collective effects of Maharishi's Transcendental Meditation and TM-Sidhi program gives clear evidence for consciousness existing not only as a localized subjective phenomenon associated with a particular nervous system, but also as an unbounded field.

The research also helps to resolve long-standing discussion on the relationship between the brain, consciousness, and quantum mechanical effects, which has carried over into the field of development of consciousness. Scientists have proposed that in higher states of consciousness, the brain has the capacity not only to detect the underlying, unbounded field, but also to stimulate it. In this theory, the brain begins to function at the quantum-mechanical level; it becomes the "quantum brain."

In the past, leading physicists and neuroscientists have suggested that brain functioning may be inherently quantum mechanical. For example, Neils Bohr, one of the founders of quantum mechanics, suggested that thought involved such small energies in the brain that it may be governed by quantum effects. Another Nobel laureate, physicist Eugene Wigner, in his work on the quantum theory of measurement, pointed to an intimate and unavoidable relationship between the quantum mechanical wave function and human consciousness.

Researchers over the years have suggested a number of models of brain functioning and quantum effects. For example, memory and information retrieval have been described in terms of quantum mechanical systems, and models of nerve transmission in terms of quantum-mechanical tunneling. More recently, Nobel laureate Sir John Eccles suggested quantum effects at the synaptic gap, the tiny space between communicating nerve cells. At the synaptic gap, tiny vesicles are released. These vesicles carry the neurotransmitter substances responsible for the transmission of information from one nerve to another. Sir Eccles' calculations indicate that the probability of a vesicle's emission from the synapse might be influenced by mental intention, similarly to the way it has been suggested that mental intention modifies a quantum wave function in quantum measurement theory. He thus suggests a means by which the mind influences the body.

The Hydrogen Atom of the Conscious Nervous System

The physicist Dr. Lawrence Domash suggests that consciousness can be considered a quantum wave function phenomenon and that pure consciousness represents a phase transition to a macroscopic quantum wave function. In developing his model, he first asks if it is possible to find what a physicist might consider the "hydrogen atom"— the simplest atomic structure—of the conscious nervous system. It must be, he says, a state of consciousness less active than ordinary waking state, yet, unlike dreaming or deep sleep, preserving the element of conscious inner awareness with minimum thought and physiological activity. He suggests that the state of pure consciousness described in the Vedic tradition is this state.

As a rationale, Dr. Domash points out that consciousness can be viewed as a "dimmer" phenomenon, rather than an on-off switch. It is capable of being decreased, as in drowsiness and deep sleep, or increased (expanded), as in pure consciousness. He suggests that the nervous system is capable of a series of phase transitions that sequentially give rise to different states of consciousness.

He says that the level of consciousness may be related to the degree of long-range spatial and temporal ordering of the brain's billions of neurons. We can think of the TM technique as a means of systematically de-exciting the nervous system as a correlate to the lower "mental temperature" produced during the practice, while preserving conscious awareness. At the level of least excitation of consciousness, a phase transition occurs in the brain to a distinct and more highly ordered state, stabilized temporally and highly correlated spatially, that gives rise to the subjective experience of "pure" consciousness.

Dr. Domash suggests that the type of phase transition occurring within the nervous system during TM is a direct result of a kind of macroscopic quantum behavior. He feels it is similar to superconductivity in metals, the remarkable phenomenon that can occur when you cool a circular bar of lead or tin to close to absolute zero (–459.67°F).

In Chapter 9, we described the Meissner Effect in superconductors to illustrate how invincible national consciousness is produced through the Maharishi Effect. Another property of superconductors is that if you apply an electrical current to one, there is no resistance, and the current will flow eternally through the circular bar. The flow of the current is frictionless, because all of the electrons are perfectly correlated with each other. Even though it is still a classical system, the bar of lead has taken on the characteristics of the quantum world. The appearance of superconductivity at much higher temperatures in certain materials is an exciting new development in this field.

Researchers have already postulated the appearance of high-temperature superconductivity in biological systems. Dr. Domash suggests that the site most appropriate to look for these quantum effects is the synapse, the same site proposed by Sir John Eccles and other scientists. Dr. Domash theorizes that during the TM technique, superconductivity causes neurons to act coherently with each other.

In this model the physiology of consciousness becomes perfectly integrated with the physiology of matter. Macroscopic quantum coherence within the nervous system can be considered a state in which the unbounded subjective properties of pure consciousness—expansion, perfect correlation, and orderliness—are manifest in the objective physiology of matter.

The Field Effects of Consciousness

Dr. John Hagelin has introduced a comprehensive new model of consciousness that greatly extends the earlier quantum mechanical theories by incorporating the most current unified quantum field theories of physics. In his model, Dr. Hagelin considers the important question of the precise nature of the field that mediates the Maharishi Effect.

The most obvious candidates for such long-range interaction are electromagnetism and gravity. As Dr. Hagelin explains, however, any conventional gravitational interaction between individuals is presumably orders of magnitude too weak to sustain long-range effects. The case for electromagnetism is also not completely satisfying, although there is some evidence that the brain may be sensitive to weak field effects. For example, researchers have found that the physiology may be sensitive to environmental AC electric fields six to seven orders of magnitude weaker than had been previously suspected.

Dr. Hagelin feels that in order to account for Yogic Flying and the Maharishi Effect, we need to go beyond conventional mechanisms and postulate an alternate theoretical framework at the level of superunification, the level of the unified field of all the laws of nature. At the Washington news conference described earlier, Dr. Hagelin presented to the journalists an excellent summary of his theory.

"Several times in this century," he said, "physicists have been surprised by the appearance of striking quantum mechanical effects on the observable, macroscopic level. For example, in superfluidity, fluids display zero viscosity and will continue to flow indefinitely once set in motion. Such phenomena appear to contradict the laws of nature, but actually they give us a glimpse of the nature of physical reality at fundamental space-time scales. Yogic Flying demonstrates on the macroscopic level the dynamics of nature's most fundamental level, the unified field.

"Only from the level of the unified field, the level of superunification at which all four fundamental forces of nature are unified, could there be that natural command over the structure of space-time geometry to support Yogic Flying. Classical theories of gravitation, theories such as Newtonian gravity and Einstein's general relativity, cannot explain Yogic Flying. However, quantum gravity can.

"Quantum gravity is a theory of gravity that ordinarily applies to the nature of physics at the scale of the unified field. This is a level of nature's functioning which is prior to classical space-time geometry. At this level, space-time geometry is dynamically generated. It is possible, through the generation of a sustained coherent influence at the level of the unified field, to modify the local curvature of space-geometry described in general relativity in such a way that the body flies up, or to the left, or forward, or in any possible direction. On the basis of currently conceivable ideas in physics, it is only through a technology of the unified field that Yogic Flying is possible."

At the time, I wondered how many members of the press would

understand this extraordinary discussion. The principles at the basis of Dr. Hagelin's explanation weren't being taught even in normal under-graduate-level physics courses. They were on the cutting edge of modern physics and truly understood by only a handful of experts. But the education of the audience did not stop there. Dr. Hagelin patiently explained in the simplest possible terms that at the level of the unified field, all aspects of natural law everywhere in the universe become infi-nitely correlated with each other.

"This means," he said, "that a delicate impulse at one point in the system can create a precipitous change throughout the entire universe. This long-range correlation explains how action on the level of the unified field can have an influence that spreads anywhere and every-where throughout the universe. In this way, the phenomenon of coher-ence spreads, neutralizing negative tendencies in the whole creation."

Since that news conference, Dr. Hagelin has elaborated extensively on these ideas and presented them to physicists at leading universities throughout the world. He points out that while we do not currently possess the calculative tools to unify the full dynamics of quantum grav-ity, the structure of space-time below the Planck scale (10^{-33} cm) appears to involve very unexpected phenomena and characteristics very similar to those of pure consciousness as described by Maharishi. Further, there are many possible mechanisms at the scale of superunification that might help explain the Extended Maharishi Effect. (For example, one possible mechanism might be "wormholes"—tunnels in the structure of space-time that enable communication at enormous distances.)

Dr. Hagelin provides us with the basic framework for formulating a field model of consciousness. It is appropriate to call this model Maharishi's field model of consciousness since it is derived from his insights and predictions. While more experimental data is needed to pro-vide a precise mathematical description of this model, we can conclude from the existing data that it must have several basic characteristics.

First, consciousness in its purest state is the unified field of natural law. Second, consciousness in its more excited states appears as a local-ized individual phenomenon, but in reality this localized consciousness is merely a particular vibrational mode of the underlying field. (As I mentioned at the beginning of the book, this completely parallels quantum field theory, in which elementary particles are described as stable vibrational modes of the underlying quantum field.) Third, when we transcend normal waking activity and experience the unified field directly, the nervous system undergoes a phase transition to a more orderly state. Fourth, during the group practice of Maharishi's Transcendental Meditation and TM-Sidhi program, this underlying field of consciousness can be stimulated in specific ways with observable effects (such as the Maharishi Effect). Fifth, we can detect and measure the field effects of consciousness using widely available sociological data.

The Power of Consciousness

How does Maharishi's TM-Sidhi program, particularly Yogic Flying, stimulate the underlying field of consciousness to create orderliness in the surroundings? During Transcendental Meditation, mental activity becomes increasingly refined until one experiences the field of pure, transcendental consciousness. The TM-Sidhi program uses specific techniques that enliven and activate transcendental consciousness and develop the habit of projecting thought and action from this simplest state of human awareness. The TM-Sidhi techniques are a natural extension of the effortless practice of the TM technique; they may be learned after a few months of TM practice.

Maharishi describes the mechanics of the TM-Sidhi program and how the mind-body relationship develops through this practice:

> In this program, human awareness identifies itself with that most wide and most powerful level of nature's functioning and starts to function from there. The purpose of the TM-Sidhi program is to consciously create activity from that level where nature performs.

> Because the state of least excitation is basic to all excited states, the mind in this state gains the upper hand. The mind becomes more basic to its own excited states, which is the body. On that level where the awareness becomes more basic to the body, the mind-body relationship has reached its climax. The ultimate relationship between mind and body is that the mind is the master of its own projections. The body is a projection of the mind, and therefore the mind can be master of the body.

The Sanskrit term *sidhi* means "perfection." Each TM-Sidhi technique is a method to develop optimal functioning—perfection—in specific functions of the mind or channels of mind-body coordination. For example, techniques are used to enhance the senses, develop virtues, and develop abilities such as being able to move through the air by mere intention. (These abilities are commonly referred to as *sidhis*.)

Maharishi's TM-Sidhi program originates in the Yog Sutras of Patanjali, one of the great teachers in the Vedic tradition. *Yog sutr* means "thread of unity." The goal of the TM-Sidhi program is to enliven specific aspects or "threads" of mind-body coordination and thus, in Maharishi's words, "weave the holistic fabric" of Unity consciousness.

In the Yog Sutras, Patanjali calls the technique to produce the Sidhi phenomena *sanyam*. Sanyam consists of the simultaneous application of three diverse modes of awareness: *dharan*, steadiness of the mind; *dhyan*, transcending; and *samadhi*, the state of pure consciousness. Maharishi's TM-Sidhi program contains a set of specific mental formulas which, when properly used through the technique of sanyam, produce predicted results and promote the rapid development of higher states of consciousness in the individual and a holistic evolutionary effect in the environment.

Maharishi emphasizes that successful performance of the TM-Sidhi program through the process of sanyam can occur only at the junction point between the active mind and silent pure consciousness. He explains that, at the point where the awareness has become so subtle as to merge with the unboundedness of pure consciousness, the term "thinking process" takes an entirely new form—it becomes one with the self-interacting dynamics of the field of pure consciousness: "One's own transcendental consciousness, functioning within itself during the TM-Sidhi program, is the unified field functioning within itself. In the TM-Sidhi program we practice that self-referral, self-interacting activity." Here, the mind is stationed at the level from where the performance of sanyam can elicit the total organizing power of the unified field to promote the desired effect.

Success in the TM-Sidhi techniques depends on the degree to which the mind has become established in the field of pure consciousness. Vedic seers thus regarded the sidhis, particularly Yogic Flying, not only as a means to develop higher states of consciousness, but also as a measure of one's level of consciousness.

This measure is far more informative than any other means of verification we have today. EEG coherence, sophisticated as it is, can give only an approximation of the brain's neurophysiological activity during higher states of consciousness, let alone a precise measure of an individual's ability to directly experience the unified field of nature's intelligence.

Earlier, we saw that there are three stages of Yogic Flying (hopping, hovering, and sustained flight), which represent progressively greater integration between the physiology and consciousness. Those practicing Maharishi's TM-Sidhi program have so far enjoyed only the first stage; this is in part, Maharishi explains, because world consciousness is still full of stress and therefore not coherent enough to support the full unfoldment of Yogic Flying.

In terms of neurophysiology, sidhis can be considered to be encoded in the genetic potential of the human nervous system. They require, however, a certain level of coherence in the nervous system, achieved through neurophysiological refinement, before this potential can be spontaneously activated.

Research has found a high level of EEG coherence during the TM-Sidhi program—especially during Yogic Flying. Dr. Orme-Johnson explains that "when one examines the EEG of a nonmeditator, one sees simple, synchronous activity in some parts of the brain and more complex, desynchronized activity elsewhere. In TM meditators one sees a high level of synchrony in the entire brain.

"Long-term TM meditators show very high levels of EEG coherence. During the Yogic Flying technique, one sees maximum coherence. Brain wave coherence also increases longitudinally. Measure the EEG of a meditator today, in three months, and again after a year, and you will see increasing coherence in the different brain areas compared with control groups. Individuals with higher levels of brain wave coherence are more creative, have higher levels of moral judgment, are more intelligent, and can assimilate information from the environment more efficiently."

Perhaps most interesting, during Yogic Flying high EEG coherence across all brain wave frequencies is seen in the midst of dynamic activity—just before the onset of the hopping phenomenon characteristic of the technique's first stage. When you examine the EEGs of the same individuals voluntarily jumping, you do not see the same results. Only Yogic Flying produces this strong brain wave coherence.

In the Yogic Flying competition described at the beginning of the chapter, medals were awarded to those who went the fastest, the highest, and the farthest in the various events. Such competitions have since become annual events around the world. But an important point Dr. Morris brought out at the first one, which participants in these events well understand, is that the real competition is not in the outer display of certain special abilities. It is rather, he said, "in generating the most delicate impulse in the unified field to accomplish Yogic Flying on the ground of the Self, the ground of pure silence, which is the unified field of natural law. The real champions are they who go most profoundly into the Self and generate most powerfully that beautiful, coherent influence on the level of the unified field which is the basis for creating coherence in world consciousness and world peace."

This powerful enlivenment of the unified field produces not only strong brain wave coherence. Subjectively, the experience is one, not of strenuous exertion, but of a tremendous upsurge of energy and bliss. Several competitors at the first Yogic Flying demonstrations were interviewed by the press afterwards, and their comments bore this out. One described his experiences as "blissful and exhilarating—you just want to go on and on." Another said, "In the finals, I felt more and more joy inside. The longer the competition went on, the deeper I felt." These are common experiences among those who practice Yogic Flying. Maharishi has explained that it is the "bubbles of bliss" arising in thousands of Yogic Flyers worldwide that have been nourishing the world from the unified level of nature's intelligence and purifying the whole of world consciousness.

The traditions of many cultures contain accounts of people who appear to have exhibited sidhis—even the ability to levitate or float. Historical descriptions of their experiences also bring out the value of bliss, or "rapture."

> When one sits in meditation, the fleshly body becomes quite shining like silk or jade. It seems difficult to remain sitting; one feels as if drawn upwards. . . . In time, one can experience it in such a way that one really floats upward.—*The Secret of the Golden Flower, A Chinese Book of Life*

> Rapture is essentially irresistible. . . . It sweeps upon you so swift and strong that you see and feel yourself being caught up in this cloud and

borne aloft as on the wings of a mighty eagle. . . . Even at times my whole body has been lifted from the ground. —St. Theresa of Avila

St. Richard, then chancellor to St. Edmund, Archbishop of Canterbury, one day softly opening the chapel door, to see why the archbishop did not come to dinner, saw him raised high in the air, with his knees bent and his arms stretched out. . . . —*The Origins of Culture*

During the seventeen years he [St. Joseph of Cupertino] remained at Grottella over seventy occasions are recorded of his levitation. . . . —Butler's *Lives of the Saints*

Inspiring as these descriptions are, in the modern era people often dismiss them as exaggerations. Also, this kind of experience has been seen as open to only a few special individuals down through the centuries. Maharishi explains that it was the coming of the scientific age that made it possible for people to once again appreciate the practical significance of Vedic wisdom to create health and world peace, and the scientifically proven benefits of the experience of Yog, or union, through the practice of Yogic Flying:

It needed a scientific age for the world to appreciate the significance of the philosophy of Yog and its practical application in creating integrated individuals, integrated nations, and an integrated world family.

Yog means union, the union of the individual awareness with the unified field of all the laws of nature in the state of transcendental consciousness. Yogic Flying demonstrates the ability of the individual to act from the unified field and enliven the total potential of natural law in all its expressions—mind, body, behavior, and environment. Yogic Flying presents in miniature the flights of galaxies in space, all unified in perfect order by natural law.

The mind-body coordination displayed by Yogic Flying shows that consciousness and its expression—the physiology—are in perfect balance. Scientific research has found maximum coherence in human brain functioning during Yogic Flying. As the coherently functioning human brain is the unit of world peace, Yogic Flying is the mechanics to make world peace a reality, and thereby bring world health, world happiness, world prosperity, a world free from suffering—Heaven on Earth in this generation.

Regular practice of the TM-Sidhi program, particularly Yogic Flying, Maharishi points out, is itself the quickest and most advanced means to eliminate the world's collective stress. As individuals practice Maharishi's TM-Sidhi program, they simultaneously further their own evolution while helping to create peace in the world. They are becoming masters of natural law, perfectly in tune with the unified field of natural law. With continued practice, they spontaneously radiate more coherent and positive influences within the environment. As Maharishi explained in his inaugural address to the first Yogic Flying competition in Washington, D.C., in 1986,

> I want to emphasize that the nature of the unified field is only evolutionary. The power of the unified field is only nourishing. Destruction is nonexistent in the unified field. This is a very important point. There is no danger of any destructive capability in the unified field. It is absolutely safe in the hands of those who know how to use it. Those knowers of the unified field, those who are practicing the TM-Sidhi program, have the skill of using the self-interacting dynamics of consciousness.
>
> They promote liveliness of the unified field in their own consciousness, and in groups they enliven the dormant self-interacting dynamics of the unified field to create harmony and an evolutionary influence in world consciousness. They promote coherence in world consciousness, and this spontaneously eliminates destructive trends and tendencies in life. Our means of establishing world peace are absolutely evolutionary, and therefore we feel absolutely safe in launching a program to create peace in our dear world family.

The key principle underlying the power of the TM-Sidhi program, and especially Yogic Flying, is that each individual, through development of coherent brain functioning, is able to directly experience and stimulate the unified field of natural law. This effect is magnified many times when a group of sufficient size practices the technique together.

Maharishi has explained that it is only from the level of the total potential of natural law, the level of the unified field, that a completely harmonious and holistic influence can be produced. He says, "The different levels of natural law have both values, creative and destructive. How they are used depends upon the level of consciousness of the user. . . . We want to produce that quality of world consciousness where destructive tendencies will simply not arise and whatever negative tendencies may exist will be extinguished."

The most important part of Maharishi's Program to Create World

Peace is the establishment of permanent groups of at least 7,000 Yogic Flyers on every continent to create coherence for the whole of world consciousness.

"What I see," he says, "is that world peace is the personal and immediate requirement of every significant man in the world today, and that means anyone who loves his life and the life of his neighbor. I invite every significant man in the world to rise to his responsibility and not postpone the creation of groups of 7,000 on earth for tomorrow. Every today is important, and every tomorrow is going to be important. We have the knowledge, and we should be able to give the gift of this knowledge to all mankind."

CHAPTER

11

THE WORLD IS MY FAMILY

HE SUN GLITTERED OFF THE CASCADING WATER OF THE Vltava River as I walked across the Charles Bridge in Prague. I couldn't help but think of the awe and wonder a young village boy must have felt on his first journey to this magnificent city. The remarkable towers of the famous St. Vitus' Cathedral sit high on the hill overlooking the ancient city, known as the "City of a Hundred Spires," one of Europe's finest jewels.

I was here at perhaps the most historic moment in the city's long history, a turning point in the balance of world power. Only a few months before, Prague had peacefully overthrown its communist rule, and now its new president was in Washington addressing the U.S. Congress. I got back to my hotel room just in time to see the live broadcast. It was a brilliant speech, leaving no question about the importance of the unbelievable turn of events that had transpired in 1989.

President Havel boldly said to millions of people listening worldwide, "Consciousness precedes physical being, and not the other way around, as the Marxists claim. . . . Without a global revolution in the sphere of human consciousness, nothing will change for better in the sphere of our being as humans." These words echoed the feelings of the people throughout all of Eastern Europe and much of the Soviet Union.

183

What had happened in Czechoslovakia was happening everywhere. With the dismantling of the Berlin Wall, the terrible fear and tension between the superpowers had rapidly begun to dissolve. Clearly, this time will be regarded as one of the greatest moments in the history of the world—when the Cold War ended and a new era of international cooperation began. It was the precursor to other events, including the end of Soviet communism and the breakup of the Soviet Union itself, that were even more astonishing, even miraculous. The march of world events starting from 1989 produced a complete phase transition.

How and why did this powerful momentum of change in the world take place in 1989 and since? Was it due to negotiations or peace treaties? There are many explanations. Numerous books have been written and will continue to be written on the subject. From the perspective of Maharishi's Vedic Science, however, the changes had little or nothing to do with peace treaties. Researchers have estimated that there have been approximately 9,000 peace treaties over the last three thousand years, each with an average life span of just eight years. From the perspective of the Vedic paradigm, the reason is simple, because it is much more fundamental: there was a dramatic change in world consciousness.

The World Peace Project of 1978 produced the first real data that revealed the power of consciousness to calm down violence in different countries. In 1979, Maharishi asked experts in the TM-Sidhi program ("Sidhas") to form groups in every country to maintain regular, large twice-daily group meditations. The scientific research on the effects of these groups and on several major peace projects conducted in subsequent years gives clear verification that it was the technology of consciousness that changed the world and established world peace in 1989.

Experimental Confirmation of the Maharishi Effect in the Middle East

One of the most striking demonstrations of reducing international conflict was conducted in Israel in the summer of 1983. This project was initiated by the Institute for Research on Consciousness and Human Development at Harvard University. The study was supported in part through a grant from the Fund for Higher Education in New York and was conducted by Dr. David Orme-Johnson, Dr. Charles

Alexander, and their co-workers.

This was a prospective study, in which certain specific results were predicted before its actual implementation. The study aimed to gather together in Jerusalem 200 people, the square root of one percent of the population of Israel, to collectively practice the Transcendental Meditation and TM-Sidhi program. Because many of the participants had professional responsibilities, the actual number of participants varied from week to week, reaching 200 during one two-week period and on several weekends. This constantly varying pattern actually enabled a more careful statistical analysis of the Extended Maharishi Effect.

Results of the study clearly demonstrated the effect: when the number of participants went up, there was a significant decrease in reported war deaths in Lebanon, a decrease in the intensity of the Lebanon war (as measured by news content analysis), a decrease in fires and automobile accidents in both Jerusalem and in Israel as a whole, and an increase in the Israeli stock market. Using a statistical procedure known as time series analysis, a clear relationship was determined between the overall quality of life in Jerusalem, Israel, and Lebanon (as measured by a composite index of many different variables) and the number of TM-Sidhi participants.

The study was submitted to one of the most prestigious and conservative journals in the field, the *Journal of Conflict Resolution*, edited at Yale University. It took more than three years before it was finally published. The editor, Dr. Bruce Russett, preceded the article with a rare editor's comment, in which he stated the following:

> The following article presents and tests a hypothesis that will strike most readers (myself included) as, to say the least, unorthodox. The hypothesis, supported by empirical tests, is that the practice of Transcendental Meditation by a relatively small group of individuals can lower the manifestations of social conflict in a much wider circle of individuals not in any contact with the meditators. This hypothesis has no place within the normal paradigm of conflict and peace research. Yet the hypothesis seems logically derived from the initial premises, and its empirical testing seems competently executed. These are the standards to which manuscripts submitted for publication in this journal are normally subjected.

In any paradigm shift, there is often a resistance between old and new ideas. It is difficult for researchers to accept a new hypothesis, especially when it so clearly conflicts with their existing ideas. This is precisely what occurred in the publication of this study. Yet the fact that it was published is an important step in the shift to the new Vedic paradigm.

A Taste of Utopia

The most ambitious and widely publicized demonstration of the effect of group practice of the Transcendental Meditation and TM-Sidhi program on world peace took place in Fairfield, Iowa, home of Maharishi International University, for three weeks at the end of 1983. This marked the first time the Maharishi Effect was tested on a global scale. The demonstration was an assembly called "A Taste of Utopia." It was announced as a global sociological experiment and was the first time in world history that more than 7,000 people—the square root of one percent of the world's population—gathered to collectively practice the TM-Sidhi program.

Prior to the assembly, a number of predictions were made, including improvements in international relations and in major world stock markets, and a worldwide decrease in crime, accidents, and illness. In each case the predictions were confirmed. The effects were so widespread that the entire phenomenon earned a new name, the Global Maharishi Effect.

For example, the World Index of international stock prices, a single measure of stock prices (the weighted average of 1,100 securities listed in the 19 most important stock exchanges in the world), had been generally going down for three weeks prior to the course. At the onset of the assembly the index began to rise, and rose steadily until the first Monday after the assembly ended, when it suddenly declined again. Eighteen of the 19 markets included in the World Index increased, 8 of the 11 largest markets in the world broke all-time records, and the U.S. market, after a long downward trend, suddenly rallied during the three weeks of the assembly. During the same three-week period in the previous five years, an average of half the markets went up and half went down.

In other areas of the study, U.S. traffic fatalities over the 1983 Christmas and New Year holiday dropped to an all-time low, even though the miles driven were at an all-time high. There were 31% fewer fatalities per mile driven than in the previous 16 years. Infectious diseases dropped by 15% in the U.S. compared with the three-week periods before and after the assembly, and by 32% compared with the mean of the same time period during the five previous years. U.S. patent applications increased 15% over the amount normally predicted by the United States Patent Office, and then decreased to normal values immediately after the assembly. (All these statistics take into account seasonal increases.) Regarding international affairs, content analysis of newspapers revealed that for the three weeks before the assembly, positive events comprised 18% of the total number of events worldwide. This percentage increased to 31% during the assembly, and then decreased to 13% afterward.

One intention of the assembly was to decrease violence in one of the most troubled areas of the world, Lebanon. In addition to the Taste of Utopia, other assemblies were held between 1983 and 1985 that had a theoretically sufficient number of TM-Sidhi experts to influence the conflict in Lebanon. Including the Taste of Utopia, there were seven assemblies in all—three in the United States, and one each in Israel, Lebanon, Yugoslavia, and the Netherlands—that were evaluated as part of long-term studies on the effects of group practice of the Transcendental Meditation and TM-Sidhi program on violence in Lebanon.

One study considered three assemblies—the Taste of Utopia and those in Yugoslavia and Lebanon. The Lebanon assembly was held in March 1984, and involved some 60 experts in the TM-Sidhi program, a number large enough to create the Maharishi Effect for Beirut and surrounding areas. The Yugoslavia assembly, of 2,000 Sidhas, was held in late April and early May, 1984. Three separate parameters were used to objectively measure the effects of these assemblies. The first two were the number of war-related injuries and war-related deaths (public statistics gathered from the Lebanese government), and the third was a peak war index compiled through content analysis of Lebanese newspapers, using raters from the three dominant factions: Christian, Moslem, and Druse.

The study extended from one month before the Taste of Utopia to one month after the Yugoslavia assembly ended, nearly 250 days. Using time series analysis the researchers found that there was a significant average drop in daily war deaths (more than 50%) and war injuries (more than 28%) during the three assemblies.

A second study, this time of all seven assemblies, replicated and extended these findings. It involved a comprehensive content analysis of events in Lebanon over an 821-day period, conducted by independent researchers at the University of Maryland. The study compared 93 experimental days (during the seven assemblies) to 718 non-experimental days. Time series analysis found that, in contrast to the non-experimental days, during the experimental days there was a 66% increase in cooperation among antagonists, a 48% decrease in the level of conflict, a 71% decrease in war-related fatalities, and a 68% reduction in war-related injuries. (These results were highly statistically significant: in statistical terms, the probability that these results might be due to chance was stated as $p < .00001$, or less than 1 in 100,000 for each variable.) Changes in temperature, holidays, and any other form of seasonality or trend were explicitly controlled for and found not to have had a significant impact on the improvements.

In July of 1985, another large assembly of 5,600 experts in the TM-Sidhi program was held in Washington, D.C. It was predicted that since the assembly was held in this important world capital, which powerfully influences not only national collective consciousness but world consciousness, less than the required number of 7,000 would be needed to produce global effects. Time series analysis showed that, as with the Taste of Utopia, there were a number of significant improvements: the Dow Jones industrial average increased significantly, the World Index of international stock prices (19 countries) increased, international conflicts decreased, infectious diseases in the U.S. decreased, fires in Washington, D.C., decreased, and U.S. patent applications increased.

One study that drew on data apart from these assemblies was especially convincing. Twelve indices of quality of life in the United States were monitored over a 23-year period from 1960 to 1983. An overall quality-of-life index was formulated using the following: (1) crime rate, (2) percentage of civil cases reaching trial, (3) infectious disease rate, (4) infant mortality, (5) suicide rate, (6) cigarette consumption per capita, (7) alcohol consumption per capita, (8) gross national product (GNP) per capita, (9) patent applications, (10) number of educational degrees conferred, (11) divorce rate, and (12) traffic fatalities. The trend of this index is clearly downward over the first part of the 23-year period, worsening rapidly after 1967 until 1975, when it reached its lowest point. It improved slightly over the next six years, until 1982, when there was a sudden increase in the rate of improvement. The index shows steady improvement after that until the end of the study.

In 1975 and 1976, the first turning point in the trend, the number of people learning the TM technique significantly increased. More than a quarter of a million people in the U.S. learned Transcendental Meditation in 1975. Interestingly, at the time Maharishi referred to 1975 as "the Dawn of the Age of Enlightenment" even though it was a time of economic and social turbulence. One year later, Maharishi introduced the TM-Sidhi program and began emphasizing the importance of gathering a sufficient number of people together to use this more advanced procedure for improving the collective health of every nation and of the world as a whole. In 1979 a permanent group of experts in the TM-Sidhi program was established in Fairfield, Iowa, associated with Maharishi International University. After several years, the group had stabilized at the required number of about 1,600 (approximately the square root of one percent of the population of North America). Since 1982, this group has collectively practiced the TM-Sidhi program, and since that time, research has shown a marked improvement in quality-of-life indices for the whole nation.

One would expect the positive influences to be most evident in Iowa itself. Of the twelve variables used in the quality-of-life index, statistics for six are available in Iowa (crime, infectious disease, infant mortality, alcohol consumption, divorce, and traffic fatalities). A separate study showed that, from 1982 to the end of the study in 1986, Iowa fared better on all of these variables than the rest of the nation.

Improved Economic and Political Indicators

One series of studies on the Maharishi Effect has focused on an economic indicator known as the misery index. These studies were conducted by Dr. Kenneth Cavanaugh, an economist and expert statistician, in collaboration with Dr. Kurleigh King, former Secretary-General of the Caribbean Community and Common Market, and most recently Governor of the Central Bank of Barbados.

The misery index, first proposed by economist Arthur Okun, is defined as the sum of the inflation rate and the unemployment rate, and is a commonly used measure of national economic performance.

Dr. Cavanaugh compared MIU's group TM-Sidhi program attendance figures, beginning with 1979 when the group first formed, with U.S. government reports on inflation and unemployment. (The MIU group program is also called the "Super Radiance" program, after superradiance in laser light, described in Chapter 9.)

Using time series analysis, he found a statistically significant relationship between high numbers practicing the Transcendental Meditation and TM-Sidhi program in Fairfield and a low misery index over an eight-year period. During this time, inflation went from 10% to 5.6%. The research suggests that about 3% of that change was directly due to the MIU Super Radiance program. The government estimates that each 1% decrease translates into savings of $32 billion ($28 billion from increased revenues and $4 billion from decreased costs in unemployment services.) These figures suggest that group practice of the TM and TM-Sidhi program saved the government some $96 billion during that period.

A different kind of study a few years ago looked at the influence of the Maharishi Effect on international relations, specifically between the United States and the Soviet Union. This study, conducted by Dr. Paul Gelderloos and Dr. Cavanaugh, provides the clearest evidence that the changes in Eastern Europe and the former Soviet Union over the past few years directly resulted from changes in collective consciousness.

The study made use of data from the Zurich Project on East-West Relations, which during that time maintained a continuous news content analysis on the relationship between the superpowers. Statements made by heads of state and other key government officials, as well as overt actions taken by each government toward the other, were scored as either hostile, neutral, or friendly. This data was tracked every month from 1979 to 1986 and compared with fluctuations in Super Radiance attendance at MIU.

The study showed that positive American statements and actions were highly correlated with increases in Super Radiance attendance over a certain threshold. Small increases foreshadowed positive actions taken by American leaders, while large increases apparently allowed the effect to be felt further away from its source in the United States, foreshadowing positive actions by Soviet leaders. In general, positive actions and statements first came from the American side and were later taken up by the Soviet Union. In other words, in the context of the times, the Super Radiance program at MIU had a powerful effect on initiating and sustaining better U.S.-Soviet relations.

To date, there are more than 40 studies on the Maharishi Effect, 25 alone on the Extended Maharishi Effect produced by group practice of the TM-Sidhi program. The scope of these studies ranges from the effects on cities and states, to those produced by a group in one country on the national life of that country, on neighboring countries, on international conflicts, and on the world as a whole. Taken together, the research provides us with experimental evidence of an effective technology to create peace in the world.

Success of Maharishi's Program to Create World Peace

In July 1986, with the first international Yogic Flying competitions, Maharishi had unveiled his Program to Create World Peace, a strong initiative to create large groups of Yogic Flyers on every continent and in every nation. He set forth several criteria for world peace: (1) friendship between the superpowers, (2) a cease-fire in the Iran-Iraq war, (3) improved international relations, and (4) an end to terrorism.

Regarding superpower relations, Maharishi explained in 1986:

> The state of world peace will be perpetual when the unified field is lived in all the different aspects of daily life of all the people on earth. For that we need to create an influence of coherence in world consciousness. Then we will see how beautifully friendly the superpowers will be to each other. The individuals of the world must create that coherence in world consciousness on the basis of which the superpowers will become such great, close friends that they will join hands in nourishing all nations.

By the summer of 1988, three of the criteria had been met. The superpowers were, indeed, becoming great friends. News reports throughout that period conveyed the increasing warmth and spirit of cooperation between Presidents Reagan and Gorbachev. Many observers felt that an end to terrorism—Maharishi's fourth criterion— was coming soon as a result of the strengthening U.S.-Soviet friendship and the continuing breakthroughs and improvements in international relations. In 1988 fewer wars were fought, worldwide military spending declined, and global arms trading leveled off. In 1989 the world experienced a dramatic turning point: a change in the political system of nearly every country in Eastern Europe, and the end of the Cold War.

Signs of rising coherence in world consciousness were apparent, as Maharishi's program was steadily implemented and the groups of Yogic Flyers in the world grew in size. (The group at Maharishi Ved Vigyan Vishwa Vidya Peeth, MIU's sister institution in Maharishi Nagar, near New Delhi, India—the Vedic University Maharishi established for Asia—was growing especially fast.) Trends of improvement could be identified in many spheres worldwide—not only political, but also economic, social, and ecological. Great strides were being made in global disarmament. Old enmities were being settled and warmer relations were developing, including new economic agreements and stronger trade ties, among many nations whose diplomatic ties in former times were mostly frozen. National and international technological priorities were becoming increasingly focused on alternative energy sources and joint initiatives to clean up and preserve the environment.

In actuality, two opposite, yet complementary trends were becoming apparent. Growing unity was seen in greater regional cooperation and a sense of increasing global unity, exemplified by the acknowledgement of growing interdependence among the members of the family of nations. Meanwhile, there was an equally strong movement towards strengthening diversity, in the increasing desire for enfranchisement among cultural minorities and the global revival of specific social, cultural, and political integrities. It was clear that the world was getting better—and equally clear that it would take a skill as great as that of nature itself to keep everything integrated: the ability to maintain perfectly unified integrity while fully satisfying all diverse trends and tendencies.

In 1989, Maharishi pointed out that it was the rising coherence in world consciousness that was creating the sudden upsurge of freedom in so many countries. He also emphasized, however, the urgent need to make the phase transition smooth by enlivening bliss in collective consciousness from the level of the unified field. Right around that time, a remarkable opportunity presented itself to employ the skilled hand of nature to strengthen unity as the basis of growing diversity, to enliven bliss as the basis of rising freedom, in the countries of Eastern Europe and the republics of the former USSR. It suddenly became possible for the first time to widely offer courses in Maharishi's technologies in these countries, and in the next two years nearly 150,000 people in that part of the world learned Transcendental Meditation.

In the spring of 1989, a delegation was invited to Moscow to address a large and influential group of physicians. Their lectures about Transcendental Meditation and Maharishi Ayur-Ved, to standing-room-only crowds, created a sensation and an astonishing demand for more knowledge, especially for immediate instruction in TM.

A few months later, a group of MIU faculty became the first team of TM teachers in the Soviet Union. They were officially invited to Armenia to offer their expertise in helping the citizenry recover from the deep shock and psychological trauma of the devastating Armenian earthquake and its aftermath. There was an immediate and almost overwhelming surge of interest in Transcendental Meditation. Huge numbers of people flocked to the TM courses the MIU faculty began giving. As the first people began to experience the deep inner peace, calm, and release from physical and emotional strain that came with transcending, word quickly spread and soon many thousands of Armenians had learned the practice. It wasn't long before more teams of MIU faculty, as well as TM teachers from other countries, were invited to come and began teaching Transcendental Meditation in Moscow, cities throughout Russia and the Ukraine, and the Baltic republics—as well as in other Eastern European countries including Hungary, Czechoslovakia, Bulgaria, and Poland.

Everywhere the response was the same: every week, hundreds of people crowding into TM courses (some coming from cities a thousand miles away), and then relating with heartwarming enthusiasm their great joy and satisfaction with their experiences during and as a result of the practice. Even more eloquent than their words was the radiant glow that appeared on so many faces, almost overnight.

Some of the stories the teachers brought back home after the project were especially poignant—particularly those about the elderly, who had struggled hard and lived through some of the most cataclysmic times in modern history. When they started practicing Transcendental Meditation, many of these people experienced an extraordinary transformation that was very moving to behold: even on the first day of learning the practice, one could see the care, worry, and fatigue slipping away from their faces, replaced by an expression of deep inner joy and happiness—perhaps for the first time in their lives. Almost without exception, TM students of all ages urged the teachers to convey to Maharishi their deep gratitude to him for making this knowledge available to them.

Now, several years later, Russian, Ukrainian, Estonian, and Armenian teachers of Transcendental Meditation are offering TM courses to their countrymen and women. Muscovite TM-Sidhas are helping support the process of peaceful change by creating coherence in national consciousness through their daily group practice. Hundreds of medical doctors have received training in Maharishi Ayur-Ved. Very fruitful scientific collaborations have developed, for example in research on Maharishi Amrit Kalash and on EEG (including the work of Dr. Nicolai Lyubimov, mentioned in Chapter 2). Maharishi Vedic University has been established in Moscow; courses on Maharishi's Vedic Management are being taught there, and the knowledge of his Vedic Science and Technology has been brought to the very farthest reaches of the former Soviet Union.

Thus the dramatic events in the former USSR and Eastern Europe in the past several years have been supported from within those very nations. The critical problems in these nations are obviously not yet resolved. Just as obviously, however, solutions cannot come from political or economic efforts alone. The key to the future for these nations is in continuing to relieve stress, develop the inner creativity of the people, and enliven the support of natural law for the whole population. In a very real sense, the meditators are the patriots of this new era.

The Transcendental Meditation organization in Russia now needs to establish its own permanent group of 7,000 Yogic Flyers. This is the hope of the future—not only to solve its critical economic, political, and social problems, but to create a beautiful quality of life for every Russian citizen. In the post–Cold War era, every country must secure its own inner integrity by increasing coherence in the collective consciousness of it people. This will create not only strong and prosperous nations, but a harmonious family of nations, like a beautiful mosaic made up of many patterns. With this will come a new style of international relations, in which the attitude of every nation toward every other nation will be, as the expression in the Vedic literature states, *Vasudhaiv kutumbakam*—"The world is my family."

CHAPTER 12

ALLIANCE WITH
THE GOVERNMENT OF NATURE

A S THE 1990'S BEGAN, THE WORLD SEEMED TO BE ON THE verge of global peace. But Maharishi commented that permanent, irreversible world peace would be possible only if at least one group of 7,000 TM-Sidhi experts was established somewhere in the world. This goal had not yet been achieved, and although improvements were seen almost everywhere, anxiety still prevailed in the world, and the state of peace in many areas seemed at best precarious and fragile—which only made clearer the need for Maharishi's programs to be quickly implemented everywhere.

In the years since the discovery of the Maharishi Effect, Maharishi has many times invited governments to establish and support a coherence creating group of 7,000 Yogic Flyers to enliven the support of natural law, solve their nation's problems and create peace for the world. In addition to direct contacts with government leaders, these offers have also sometimes been made through full- or double-page announcements in the major newspapers and magazines of the world, with headlines such as "Maharishi Offers Governments . . ." or "Governments Invited . . ."

The theme of these invitations in recent years has been "Alliance with Nature's Government." The headline of one such announcement in the early 1990s read, "Unified Field Science and Technology Offers the Balance of Power in the World to Any Government." Its main point, summarized in several paragraphs at the top, is worth quoting at length, as it is representative of Maharishi's basic message to governments throughout the years:

> Half a century ago, Einstein brought to the attention of President Roosevelt the enormous destructive potential available at the nuclear level of natural law. "Hiroshima" was the result, and the balance of power in the world fell into the hands of the destroyer.
>
> Today, Maharishi is offering the balance of power in the world to any government through the use of the indomitable, nourishing power of natural law available in the unified field of all the laws of nature.
>
> As the unified field is the most basic field of natural law, the unified field technology is the most powerful techology—much more powerful than the electronic and nuclear technologies.
>
> Any government which uses the Maharishi Technology of the Unified Field [the TM and TM-Sidhi program] will hold the balance of power in the world and will have the ability to nourish every nation and will enjoy the guiding role—the parental role—in the family of nations.
>
> For decades the world had been under an umbrella of fear and suppression due to the balance of power resting in the hands of those having the maximum ability to destroy.
>
> Today, however, with the rise of the Maharishi Effect (coherence) in world consciousness brought about by the Maharishi Technology of the Unified Field, the destructive capabilities of the superpowers have been subdued and this has created the dawn of a new era of freedom in the world.
>
> Now time demands that governments succeed in handling this global rise of freedom and guide it in the evolutionary direction, so that everyone and every nation in the world realizes the supreme goal of freedom—Heaven on Earth.
>
> For this, there is only one choice—take recourse to the nourishing, evolutionary power of natural law through the Maharishi Technology of the Unified Field and thereby come into alliance with nature's government.
>
> By establishing a group of 7,000 people professionally engaged in the Maharishi Technology of the Unified Field, any one government can ensure that all political, economic, social, and religious trends in the family of nations are always positive, progressive, and peaceful.

The announcement also featured the following statement from Maharishi, which pointedly expressed both the utter simplicity of his solution to the world's problems, and his impatience with the world's intelligentsia for not having widely adopted it thus far: "It must be easy for anyone with the slightest intelligence to understand that if the unified field of natural law—the total value of all the laws of nature—could be accessible to anyone, nothing will be impossible for him at any time."

The fluctuations in the world situation have sometimes created great urgency in these offers. In October 1990, an announcement appeared, headlined "His Holiness Maharishi Mahesh Yogi Offers Solution to the Gulf Crisis—Calls for a Group of 7,000 Yogic Flyers Anywhere in the World—Foresees End to Tensions within One Week if His Program is Adopted." At that time, Maharishi also spoke by conference telephone with journalists all over North America. He pointed out that peace would never come through political alliances. And, he said, everyone knows that what happened to Kuwait could happen to anyone or any country at any time. The countries that had not responded to his earlier offer of "Alliance with Nature's Government" were now assembled in the Gulf. This time, he appealed not just to governments but directly to the people of the world, to create a group of 7,000 to "provide security for every nation and . . . create a united world family."

Maharishi explained that the evolutionary power of natural law enlivened during his Transcendental Meditation and TM-Sidhi program automatically increase the positivity and coherence in the whole of world consciousness, "and this brings invincibility, not just to one nation, but to all nations simultaneously." He compared the result that could be expected in the Middle East to what had already happened to the rivalry of the superpowers: "Neither side will be defeated. Both sides will come out victorious and there will be peace." He promised that the invincible force of natural law generated by the group of 7,000 would not allow the wealthy nations to continue to "make weapons and rule the world through fear of destruction. These days will soon be over."

As Maharishi explained his offer to the press, again it boiled down to a stunningly simple logic: "If the intelligence of nature can keep the big universe growing all the time in perfect orderliness, why can't this little world of ours be administered from that same level of intelligence? By awakening nature's intelligence during TM, it is completely possible to live in perfect peace and perfect national and international relations."

In January 1991, as the negotiations in the Gulf were breaking down, Maharishi appealed directly to President Bush in a message that appeared in the *Washington Post*, which said in part: "Military action and destruction in the Gulf will not stop the birth of aggression in the world in the future. Please note that our program—7,000 Yogic Flyers—will end once and for all the birth of aggression in the world. . . . We are urging this because this would prove to be a permanent solution and would make world consciousness integrated and world peace irreversible."

As we know, governments did not respond to Maharishi's appeal, and the Gulf crisis became the Gulf war. From one point of view, the superior weaponry and technological wizardry of the U.S. and its allies were responsible for winning the war with astounding swiftness. But even that power was not enough to resolve the chaos, terrible ecological damage, and human suffering in the war's aftermath. And a year after the war's conclusion, even its technological successes were being called into question.

When governments have not responded directly to his invitations, Maharishi has understood this as part of the mechanics described in his own philosophy of government, which states that governments are only an "innocent mirror" of collective consciousness. Government leaders—however much they as individuals may want to act for the good of the nation—can only express in their thinking and behavior the level of coherence in collective consciousness. They cannot act for positivity unless collective consciousness is positive. If collective consciousness is full of turbulence and negativity, then the actions of political leaders will only express that.

Ironically, this has sometimes produced a "catch-22" situation, in which the leaders of the very countries that most badly need coherence may actually be aware of, and even interested in, adopting Maharishi's programs in order to create it. However, they have been prevented from acting in favor of complete positivity by the very turbulence in collective consciousness that they seek to amend. Maharishi's offers to governments have been in one sense a means of testing the level of coherence in collective consciousness.

I have always marveled at and appreciated Maharishi's boldness all these years in proclaiming his message of global peace and invincibility for every nation. He began in 1957, one man alone. He had taught Transcendental Meditation to thousands of people across a wide spectrum of ages, educational and cultural backgrounds, and it worked for everyone. On that basis Maharishi had one goal—to bring peace and happiness to every single person in the world. He was prepared to personally teach every person if that was necessary. With this simple yet powerful resolution he traveled the world over, and wherever he went people were drawn to the possibility of a better life, came forward to learn Transcendental Meditation, and helped him accomplish his great plan.

Over the years, a number of governments have been quietly looking into Maharishi's programs and adopting them, for example in their health care, educational, and prison systems. Now, more and more governments are openly acknowledging the validity of these programs as the solution to many of their countries' problems, and are formally requesting their widespread implementation.

In the last few years there has also been increasing interest in Maharishi's knowledge from the side of the news media. When he announced his solution to the Gulf crisis, the world media responded with unprecedented coverage, including many press interviews with him. This interest has continued nearly unabated.

Maharishi has always made clear that irrespective of any actions by governments to adopt his programs and technologies on a wide scale, coherence is rising in world consciousness—as a result of the sheer numbers of people in the world who are practicing his Transcendental Meditation and TM-Sidhi program (as this book goes to press, over four million meditators worldwide). This is the way out of the "catch-22" dilemma, and it is the fruit of the many courses, assemblies, and initiatives to teach Transcendental Meditation that have been organized every year under Maharishi's inspiration through the various branches of his worldwide movement. He gives credit for the dawn of world peace, the rise of freedom, and all the growing positive trends to these assemblies; to the permanent groups of Yogic Flyers that have been established at MIU and elsewhere; and to the millions of TM meditators and Sidhas around the world who have every day been quietly creating orderliness in their own brain physiology and radiating that coherence into their surroundings.

At the time of the Gulf war, it had seemed that the war came because of a failure to prevent it by creating a group of 7,000 Yogic Flyers. Yet a year later, in light of the dramatic political changes in the USSR, it was clear that if the United States and the USSR had still been enemies in January 1991, the Gulf war might well have become World War III. As it was, the war began only after a remarkable display of world unity and great efforts to avoid war. Although the war deaths on either side of the conflict were deplorable, considering the enormous danger of global conflict with all the great powers involved, and compared to the almost unimaginable level of destruction of the first two world wars, it ended with comparatively little bloodshed. The fighting was not able to spread; the potential world war did not develop; and this indicated that peacefulness had grown in the world. At the same time, the continuing volatile political situation in the Gulf and in the Balkans indicates just as strongly the critical need to create even greater coherence in the collective consciousness of the entire world.

The Constitution of the Universe

Maharishi called 1991 his year of "Support of Nature's Government." Towards the end of the year, two things happened that Maharishi felt came as the gifts, or fruits, of that year. The group of Yogic Flyers at Maharishi Ved Vigyan Vishwa Vidya Peeth in India, the land of the Ved, became the first permanent group of 7,000 in the world.

The second gift, which Maharishi considers of even greater significance, was his discovery of the Constitution of the Universe, which was announced in several of the world's largest newspapers. Maharishi's discovery locates the single, universal source of all orderliness in nature in the self-interacting field of pure intelligence at the basis of all the diverse laws of nature in the universe. I mentioned briefly in Chapter 1 the rationale behind Maharishi's term: just as the constitution of any nation represents the basis of all the laws governing that nation, the laws governing the self-interacting dynamics of the field of pure intelligence can therefore be called the Constitution of the Universe, the ultimate source of order and harmony displayed throughout the cosmos.

In Maharishi's Vedic Science and Technology, these laws are found in the eternal, self-interacting dynamics of consciousness knowing itself, and are embodied in the structure of the Rik Ved, the most fundamental aspect of the Vedic literature. In modern physics, an identical description is found of the laws governing the unified field of all the laws of nature. (In Chapter 14, we will explore in more detail the structure of the Constitution of the Universe as found in the Rik Ved and in modern physics.)

In a global telecast at the time, Maharishi explained that the Constitution of the Universe is lively on the level of the transcendental consciousness of everyone. Therefore everyone can identify and own this level of cosmic law simply and effortlessly through Maharishi's Transcendental Meditation and TM-Sidhi program. During TM-Sidhi Yogic Flying, one "enlivens the authority of cosmic law—its absolute order and harmony—in every impulse of his thought, speech, and behavior."

"We have been teaching these simple programs for 34 years, and millions of people report greater support of nature—they begin to feel better in all areas of their lives," Maharishi said. "The time has now come for everyone—every individual, group, and nation—to live this basic reality, the Constitution of the Universe, the home of all the laws of nature. It will be a beautiful time, when the reality of life will belong to everyone."

Maharishi urged all government leaders to "incorporate the Constitution of the Universe into the life of your nations, come out of weaknesses, and satisfy everyone." The Constitution of the Universe, he said, is the constitution of nature's government; governments should look to nature's government for an ideal system of administration. "Nature's government administers the infinite diversity of the universe with perfect order and without a problem," he said. "For a national government to succeed its constitution must be aligned with the constitution of nature's government—the Constitution of the Universe."

Maharishi explained that a government will succeed when it is able to satisfy everyone in the country—majority and minority alike. The only government capable of doing this is nature's government, which "spontaneously brings satisfaction to everyone because it promotes all the innumerable, diverse tendencies of life in the evolutionary direction."

When a nation provides in its constitution for a permanent group of 7,000 experts practicing his Transcendental Meditation and TM-Sidhi program together in one place, he said, its government will be "on par with the government of nature and thereby enjoy problem-free administration. Governments now have a choice: adopt the constitution of nature's government or continue to struggle with problems." He emphasized that a government does not need to change its constitution; it need only add a provision ensuring a permanent group of 7,000.

Historical Failure of Governments to Create an Ideal Society

As world consciousness rises, the people of many countries are renewing principles that they hope will promote life in freedom, happiness, prosperity, and security. Their leaders are drafting new constitutions to embody these principles. As they do this, they are looking to the constitutions of other countries. However, Maharishi points out, "These leaders will find that no government has succeeded in creating an ideal society, because no constitution has proven capable of satisfying everyone in the nation. This is true of every system of government, including democracy. No constitution in the world today is really worth copying.

"Governments have always assumed that everyone in the nation cannot be satisfied," Maharishi said. "Therefore, constitutions and laws were framed to satisfy only the majority. But this principle—the basic principle of democratic government—was self-defeating. The democratic system, which allows opposition to the decisions of the majority, will it ever be able to maintain law and order in society? This is for the experienced politicians to decide."

For successful administration, a national constitution must do much more than merely set forth laws by which a person should behave and sanctions by which a person should be punished for violating those laws, Maharishi said. "The constitution must ensure that every citizen is satisfied and therefore spontaneously abides by the law—both natural law and national law." For a national government to satisfy everyone, its constitution must be rooted in natural law—the constitution of nature's government. Maharishi's Transcendental Meditation and TM-Sidhi program accomplishes this by enlivening the unified field of natural law in both individual and national consciousness.

"Throughout the ages, the history of government has been a history of failure," Maharishi said. "Now in this scientific age, that tradition can be reverted back to success. The pendulum of administration has reached its supremely deplorable state. The time has come for it to return and make the administration of every government worthy of its name. The complete knowledge of the Constitution of the Universe is now available. I invite the politicians of the world to receive training in the Constitution of the Universe and apply this knowledge in their countries. The result will be satisfaction for every citizen, a problem-free administration for the government, and peace in the family of nations."

The Constitution of the Universe is the greatest discovery of the scientific age, because it gives mankind the timely knowledge of natural law which alone is competent to eliminate all problems and raise life everywhere on earth to perfection. It has come at a time of global transformation. Current systems of politics, economics, and religion are proving incompetent to solve the world's problems and satisfy all peoples. This, in Maharishi's view, is essentially a failure of education, which does not train people to think and act spontaneously in accord with natural law.

"The study of man-made law in today's universities has not made people law-abiding in any country," Maharishi said. "People everywhere have been violating natural law and creating stress in world consciousness. This stress spontaneously breaks out as wars, crime, illness, and everything else that threatens the security of life."

Crime in the United States:
The Need for Administration through Natural Law

The failure of government to administer properly—that is, to prevent its people from violating natural law—is nowhere more prevalent than in the United States. With the dissolution of the USSR, there is one superpower in the world. All countries now look to the United

States as the most powerful nation. Yet the U.S. is still troubled with crime, disease, and social turbulence. President Clinton's inauguration was a time of celebration and renewed hope for the future, yet he himself noted at the time that the problems of our nation transcend and exceed the comprehension of any human being.

The worst problem in America is crime. There is a feeling of desperation among our citizens at the failure to control it. In 1992 in the United States, 1.1 million people were in prison—one out of every 200 people. If crime continues to rise at the current rate, five percent of the population will be in prison by the year 2000. In 1992 the Los Angeles riots shook the nation to its core and brought to the forefront of public attention the grave situation in the inner cities.

The U.S. government is well aware of the research on Transcendental Meditation, Maharishi Ayur-Ved, and the Maharishi Effect. Even a handful of the studies showing reduced crime in cities through the Maharishi Effect, lower recidivism among prison inmates practicing TM, 50% reduced health care usage among TM meditators in general, and reduced blood pressure among elderly urban African Americans give compelling evidence and strong arguments for the ability of these technologies to solve major national problems. And with the nation and the world still filled with anxiety for the future, it only makes sense to use the technique that research shows is most effective at reducing anxiety.

The rising coherence in collective consciousness created by U.S. meditators and the coherence creating group at MIU will continue to support progressive trends in national life, for example the growing national focus on health and the environment. However, to create the ground for perfect positivity in every corner of the nation, and in every influence of the nation in its international affairs, it needs to be firmly established in administration through natural law.

Recently, Maharishi has spoken of the danger of U.S. government leaders making decisions that crucially affect the nation and the world in the atmosphere of crime prevalent in Washington, D.C., which has the nation's highest homicide rate and is one of the most crime-ridden capitals in the world. Every government decision is shaped by the influence of crime and fear in the collective consciousness.

Now is clearly the time for Maharishi's practical, proven technologies, which are so simple, so cost-effective, and simply so effective, to be widely adopted in the United States. When the nation is crying out, not to use a solution that is so promising and so easy to implement is irresponsible, even shameful. The simplest way to implement this solution is for the government to align its constitution with the Constitution of the Universe—by establishing and supporting at least one group of 7,000 Yogic Flyers anywhere in the U.S.

Maharishi has recently emphasized this theme, giving it the title "A Group for a Government." The concept has developed to establish, in addition to one 7,000 group, a special group of at least 2,000 Vedic pandits—Yogic Flying experts from India—in Washington, D.C. This group will ensure that the intelligence of nature which administers the entire universe will support every aspect of national life through the decisions of the government.

The need for such a group is clear. And yet the experience of so many years shows us that to expect the leaders of a society pervaded by stress, fear, and crime to adopt a powerful program to eliminate crime is to ask the impossible. Our government leaders, despite their best intentions, cannot eliminate problems. Thus the responsibility for establishing these groups lies with the people of the nation. We have the chance right now to create a total transformation in America and the world to administration through natural law. This will bring alliance with the government of nature and, as a result, the complete support of natural law to all governmental activities; it will simultaneously resolve all the thorny issues and seemingly ineradicable problems of crime, economic woes, and rising health care costs, to name only a few. Most of all, it will give the most valuable support the United States can possible give—far beyond negotiations or any show of arms and military might—to the establishment of irreversible world peace.

Maharishi's Master Plan to Create Heaven on Earth

Maharishi's goal now is to quickly establish several more 7,000 groups as as soon as possible, to stabilize the growing positivity in world consciousness, prevent jerks and jolts in the current phase transition to an ideal world, alleviate the remaining areas of violence, and make world peace permanent. Based on the first group in India, 7,000 will soon be established in the United States at MIU; with similar groups being established in Russia and in Holland, these groups in all parts of the globe will, in Maharishi's words, "wrap the world in coherence and peace."

In Maharishi's view, however, world peace is not enough. Peace is not just the absence of war. For Maharishi, establishing permanent, irreversible world peace is only the beginning. The effect of having several permanent groups of 7,000, he has said many times, will be not only world peace, but a quality of life for everyone on earth so beautiful that it could only be called "heavenly."

Records of Vedic civilization describe a time of peace so profound and long-lasting that it was referred to as "Heaven on Earth." Since Maharishi first came out from the Himalayas in 1957 to teach Transcendental Meditation, the goal of all his programs has always been to create Heaven on Earth once again, in this generation.

Through the technologies of consciousness Maharishi has brought to light from the Vedic literature, many age-old aspirations can be realized in this generation. In place of fear, hatred, disease, misery, and poverty, Maharishi has offered a very real way to create unlimited peace and fulfillment. In the past few years he has structured a comprehensive plan delineating the steps necessary to achieve perfection of inner and outer life in the world. It is set forth in a 1,500-page book, *Maharishi's Master Plan to Create Heaven on Earth*.

Maharishi has described Heaven on Earth as being characterized by long life in perfect health, economic prosperity, agricultural abundance, environmental balance, cultural integrity, and world peace. Every nation will spontaneously radiate a nourishing influence to every other nation, the family of nations will be harmonious, and the entire world will be a beautiful mosaic of different cultures.

The result will be that each individual awareness will encompass and own the whole of world consciousness. We will each know that we are the microcosm of the macrocosm. This is the true meaning of "the world is my family."

Heaven on Earth means living two hundred percent of life—one hundred percent of the inner value and one hundred percent of the outer value. As the inner value of life grows with the development of higher states of consciousness, it will naturally glorify the outer aspects of life. The profound knowledge of the Vedic paradigm will ensure that on every level of life, everyone will enjoy the "physiology of Heaven on Earth." This means: an enlightened society made up of individuals who experience the self-interacting dynamics of the Ved as the inner dynamics of their own nature; whose brain physiologies and nervous systems function in complete coherence.

Once again, groups of 7,000 are an important part of Maharishi's plan to create Heaven on Earth through complete education—education that will train people to think and act in accord with natural law. Maharishi's Vedic Science and Technology provides what has been lacking in education throughout the world—complete knowledge of the knower, which includes the total potential of natural law in transcendental consciousness. Maharishi contrasts this complete, Vedic Science based education with education based on modern science: "Modern civilization is proving to be uncivilized. Human rights are violated and human dignity is shadowed. This is because modern science provides only fragmented knowledge, knowledge of isolated laws of nature." He emphasizes that the complete wisdom of life can be lived easily by everyone because the complete field of knowledge is available in transcendental consciousness—pure consciousness, the simplest state of everyone's own awareness.

We don't normally think of education as being a physiological process, yet scientific research has shown us that education has a profound effect on the physiology. Our brains are not static, but extremely dynamic. What happens if we deprive the brain of the experience of transcendental consciousness, because our educational system does not consider it to be an important and necessary element in the curriculum? We deprive the individual and society of the very mechanisms by which full human development, and thus world peace, can be achieved.

By including Maharishi's Vedic Science and Technology in our educational system, we automatically provide every individual with the knowledge and experience of how to develop higher states of consciousness and, as a by-product, create world peace. Maharishi describes the outcome of such an education as "the fruit of all knowledge"—a mistake-free life lived spontaneously in accord with all the laws of nature.

Maharishi Vedic Universities:
Natural Law Based Education

Maharishi Vedic Universities, Colleges, and Schools are being founded and soon will offer this knowledge all over the world. Curricula for training teachers at existing universities have been developed, so that Maharishi's program of research in human consciousness can be part of every field of study in all countries. Maharishi Ayur-Ved Health Education Centers are also being widely established. "Now, with the programs of my Vedic Science," Maharishi has recently said, "students will directly experience the Constitution of the Universe. They will open their awareness to deeper levels of natural law, enlivening its full potential to promote lawful trends everywhere."

The goals of the educational system at Maharishi International University, which is a model of Vedic Science based education, are, in the words of MIU President Dr. Bevan Morris, "that every person on earth, from the beginning of student life through their whole life, is a student of consciousness. They gain knowledge of consciousness through research and study of knowledge; they gain higher states of consciousness, enjoy what they learn, and develop their full creative genius. They enjoy the organizing power of nature's intelligence, which is managing the galaxies and flooding through everything, so that support of nature raises their life to a heavenly level. They live the fruit of all knowledge, enjoying complete success, in their individual personal life, in their professional life, and in what they contribute to the life of the whole nation."

The introduction of Maharishi's Vedic Science and Technology into educational systems everywhere is therefore the key to achieving Heaven on Earth. As Maharishi explains, "The time demands a new knowledge. We have that knowledge in my Vedic Science, which is capable of creating Heaven on Earth—all good everywhere and non-good nowhere."

This is the promise of utopia, which has long been sought and never found. I believe that our age is destined for a different outcome. A utopian future is dawning. It began with the first demonstration that it is possible to create world peace.

But isn't utopia just a mere fancy? How is it possible to think of such a state when the long history of the human race—and its current condition—is replete with war, disease, ignorance, and poverty?

The history of the world shows that progress has always followed in the footsteps of those who dared to show imagination, who had the courage and conviction to do what they knew was right. Many of these leaders—especially in the field of knowledge—had great insights into the nature of life. They saw what everyone else saw, but in a totally new light. Copernicus observed the sun rising and setting every day, but concluded that the sun didn't move at all; it was the earth that moved around the sun. Despite great resistance from scientists, religious leaders, and others, he was eventually proved correct.

Historically it has been assumed that what cannot be conceived intellectually has no validity. This assumption has now been proved false. The accepted limits of our knowledge have been superseded again and again. And as we grow in knowledge, the world takes on new dimensions; we begin to envision greater and greater possibilities. Things considered impossible for centuries become not only possible but real. If in 1850 you told a man in New York that he could step inside a container and appear in California three hours later, he'd have said you were crazy. Yet today we not only accept airplane travel as real, we also accept that we can fly to the moon and send spacecraft to other galaxies.

Ultimately, what makes the "impossible" possible is knowledge. If we know the laws of gravity and jet propulsion, we can create ships that fly. Whatever laws of nature we know, we can create practical applications for them in our daily lives.

The great genius of the Vedic tradition, which Maharishi embodies, is that it locates the source of all the laws of nature, the source of all knowledge, in the simplest form of human awareness—pure consciousness. When we experience pure consciousness, we enliven this field of all possibilities. When we stabilize pure consciousness as a permanent reality, then literally anything is possible.

Further, the knowledge of pure consciousness is not gained on an intellectual level. It occurs experientially. It occurs automatically, without effort, using a simple technology. This is one of Maharishi's greatest contributions. We don't have to know intellectually all the laws of nature; we just effortlessly experience their source within our own awareness and automatically gain their support. As Maharishi points out, the apple fell, and Newton formulated his law of gravity. The understanding of Newton's law, however, is not necessary in order to make an apple pie and enjoy it. Anyone can switch on and enjoy TV, radio, and electricity without having to know Maxwell's equations. Theoretical knowledge of natural law is a luxury, not a requirement for enjoying the support of natural law in daily life.

Just by enlivening the unified field, the deepest level of natural law, within our own consciousness and by coming together to enliven it even more powerfully in groups, we can create a permanent effect on world conditions. In the past, visions of utopia have been based primarily on partial, fragmented knowledge of the laws of nature. Maharishi's vision of Heaven on Earth is based on complete knowledge, and is applied through simple inner technologies of consciousness that are thousands of years old. By using these technologies, we sow the seeds of world peace. Just as, with the right nurturing, the seeds of a garden bring forth their first shoots, the seeds of world peace and of Heaven on Earth—properly planted and supported by the quiet, indomitable force of nature—will inevitably blossom.

PART 4

THE PHYSIOLOGY
OF THE UNIVERSE

CHAPTER 13

MAHARISHI'S VEDIC SCIENCE AND TECHNOLOGY: THE SCIENCE OF VED

THE STEAM ROSE OFF THE GROUND ON THE HOT PLAINS of India. In the distance, the rumble of an occasional jet making its final approach to Delhi airport could be heard. Maharishi sat outside a small gazebo in the bright moonlight, in the company of an extraordinary group of Indian pandits and scholars. It was a scene that could well have taken place several millennia ago—except for a few Western scientists in the audience, the twentieth century hardly intruded.

"Man is not just a mass of cells," Maharishi explained. "In his simplest, most refined state of consciousness, man is the total potential of natural law, the field of pure potentiality, the *Ved*." The true meaning of the word Ved, he said, is not a collection of books from ancient India, as is commonly assumed by most Western and Eastern scholars. It is something entirely different. "Ved means *knowledge*," Maharishi said, "complete knowledge, inclusive of all life." He continued, "The Ved is present at every point in creation; it is the underlying unified field of pure knowledge, of pure consciousness, from which all diversity emerges."

I thought of the sharp contrast between this expanded vision of Maharishi's Vedic Science and our immature, localized vision of modern classical science, which does indeed see the body as a mass of cells that somehow has had life breathed into it. Certainly modern science has desired to embrace the essence of life—to touch both the very small and the very large. In this search for knowledge, however, it has adopted an objective methodology that obstructs its ability to see into the deepest subjective realms of consciousness. Maharishi's Vedic Science offers a knowledge and methodology that brings fulfillment to modern science; it sees the human body as the microcosm of the macrocosm—the universe—in which all the dynamics of nature are expressed.

The Science of Ved

"Dynamism of galaxies, stars and everything in the universe is the expression of the quiet brilliant light of intelligence of natural law," Maharishi has recently written. "Natural law ever awake within everything is the light of life that administers all life with perfect orderliness." Maharishi's Vedic Science is the science that gives complete knowledge of the "quiet brilliant light of intelligence of natural law," "ever awake within everything" throughout the universe.

We want now to look more closely into Maharishi's Vedic Science and Technology, so that we can understand the greatness of this supreme science and its very practical implications for improving life on earth. Maharishi defines his Vedic Science in many ways; his primary definition is "the science of Ved."

This field of knowledge has been formulated by Maharishi on the basis of two things: the experience of pure consciousness through the Transcendental Meditation and TM-Sidhi program, and the complete theoretical and practical knowledge of the Ved, available in the Vedic literature.

First, here is Maharishi commenting on the difference between his Vedic Science and modern science:

Vedic Science is a complete science, which extends and fulfills the objective approach of modern science by incorporating the knower and the process of knowing into the field of investigation. It provides a complete and comprehensive knowledge of the unified field of all the laws of nature, which can be described as the unified state of the knower, the known, and the process of knowing.

The equations of quantum field theory can describe some of the attributes of the unified field of natural law. But only the human mind can directly experience the unified field, the basis of both matter and awareness, as the field of pure, unbounded subjectivity deep within. On that level, the totality of natural law—the Ved—can be directly experienced as the unified state of knower, process of knowing, and known.

Note Maharishi's words at the beginning of this chapter, that "Ved means knowledge, complete knowledge." On this basis he also defines Vedic Science as "the science of knowledge." He has further explained that "knowledge results from the coming together of the knower, the process of knowing, and the object of knowing," and thus another definition of his Vedic Science is "the science of the unified field [unified state] of knower, knowing, and known."

We saw in Chapter 2 that the basic level of natural law in creation, which physicists refer to as the unified field of all the laws of nature, is known in Maharishi's Vedic Science as the field of pure consciousness—an infinite field of pure intelligence or pure wakefulness—consciousness fully awake within itself, which knows itself and nothing else. We saw that, as pure consciousness knows itself, the self-referral nature of this unbounded ocean of consciousness, this unified wholeness, produces an apparent state of diversity involving three different aspects: knower, process of knowing, and known—or, in the language of Maharishi's Vedic Science, Rishi, Devata, and Chhandas. The unified state, or Samhita, of Rishi, Devata, and Chhandas constitutes the three-in-one structure of pure consciousness, the starting point of its self-interacting dynamics and the seeds of all the diversity of the universe. Thus Maharishi's Vedic Science is also "the science of consciousness."

We also saw earlier that as the self-interacting dynamics of pure consciousness continues, innumerable permutations and combinations of the interplay among Samhita, Rishi, Devata, and Chhandas values arise as countless transformations, or fluctuations, within the sea of consciousness. These transformations unfold in a precise, perfectly orderly sequence. It is this sequential unfoldment, Maharishi explains—the mechanics of transformation of unity into diversity—that forms the fundamental processes of creation. These fundamental rules of transformation are repeatedly seen at every level of creation.

Through these mechanics are created all the laws of nature that structure and govern the diverse forms and phenomena in the entire universe. It is this fundamental structure of natural law unfolding within pure consciousness, and creating the universe, that is the Ved.

Maharishi describes how the unity of pure consciousness administers the diversity of creation: "The unbounded field of pure intelligence, . . . fully awake in its pure singularity, remaining self-referral, administers itself through its infinite organizing power . . . and thereby administers all its expressions—the infinite diversity of the universe—with perfect orderliness." To illustrate this point, he often refers to a verse from the Bhagavad Gita, one of the important aspects of the Vedic literature:

> *Prakritim svam avashtabhya*
> *visrijami punah punah*
>   (Bhagavad Gita 9.8)
>
> Taking recourse to my own self-referral nature,
> I create again and again.

Thus, Maharishi explains that his Vedic Science is "the science of unity and diversity at the same time": "It is the science of unity because of Samhita—togetherness—which is the unified field, and it is the science of diversity, due to the three qualities of Rishi, Devata, and Chhandas within the structure of Samhita."

Because it is the science of unity and diversity at the same time, Maharishi ultimately defines his Vedic Science as "the science of everything": "It is the science of singularity, the self-referral subjectivity, and also it is the science of objectivity, which is nothing other than the expression of subjectivity; at the same time it is the science of transformation; it is the science of self-referral dynamics of creation. It is the science of eternal dynamism at the basis of creation."

Finally, Maharishi concludes that his Vedic Science, "being the science of everything, can be defined in terms of anything and everything." The definition of his Vedic Science, he explains, "is really beyond words due to the limitations of language and the limitless, all-encompassing nature of pure knowledge, the Ved—transcendental consciousness and the infinite range of its organizing power." It is "a perfect science which transcends intellect and transcends all expressions."

216

The Ved and the Vedic Literature: Script of the
Primordial Sounds of Nature's Intelligence

From these definitions, we can see that Maharishi's Vedic Science is no ordinary science. In Maharishi's terms, its scope "covers the whole field of Ved, and its expression, the universe." It covers "all knowledge about everything in the universe." As DNA is to the body, the Ved is to the universe. In this sense we can consider the Ved as "the physiology of the universe." Now we want to explore more deeply the physiology of the universe, the Ved itself, which, like DNA, underlies and creates all the expressed levels of manifest existence.

In Chapter 6, I discussed briefly the primordial sounds of the Ved. Maharishi describes how these primordial sounds arise from the "hum" of the vibration produced by the self-interacting dynamics of pure consciousness. The fluctuations within pure consciousness, produced by the mechanics of transformation among Rishi, Devata, and Chhandas, express different frequencies of self-interaction, which are frequencies of sound. This is what Maharishi refers to as "the language of nature," the "whisper" of the unified field of natural law to itself.

I want to introduce a new term from Maharishi's Vedic Science that expresses this concept. As the laws of nature unfold and eventually create all the material forms and phenomena of creation, they are displayed as *shruti*. Shruti refers to the sound value of the expressions of pure knowledge, the Ved and the Vedic literature, as they unfold from within pure consciousness. Maharishi defines shruti as "vibrancy of intelligence in the form of sound generated by the self-referral dynamics of consciousness." A little further on we will look in detail at the very first sounds of the Ved as it begins to unfold, and the specific mechanics of natural law these sounds express.

Maharishi explains that the most fundamental aspect of the Vedic literature is the Rik Ved, which expresses the totality of natural law. Rik Ved is the first of the four principal Vedas; the other three are Sam Ved, Yajur-Ved, and Atharv Ved. The Vedic literature comprises these four, together with all the subsequent sections that constitute what Maharishi describes as the major "branches" and "limbs" of Vedic knowledge. In Maharishi's explanation, Vedic literature displays the complete sequence of unfoldment of natural law from its source in pure consciousness, through all its increasingly more concrete expressions in every area of individual life—mind, body, and behavior—and to its fulfillment in all these areas and in the life of the entire universe.

Maharishi describes the four Vedas as "a beautiful, sequentially available script of nature in its own unmanifest state, eternally functioning within itself and, on that basis of self-interaction, creating the whole universe and governing it." And yet this simple and beautiful structure of natural law has been greatly misunderstood.

"The principal misunderstanding of the Vedas," Maharishi explains, "is that they are books or objects to be known or studied. The Vedas are *Apaurusheya*—that is, not created by individual minds, not even created by enlightened minds." Maharishi explains that the Sanskrit term Apaurusheya means "uncreated." The Vedas, he says, are the "fundamental seeds of intelligence" from which all natural laws spring; they are the dynamic impulses of natural law which make up the fabric of the unified field. They existed before space and time, they are eternal and non-changing. Maharishi describes further, "They are non-individual, existing on the level of the self-interacting dynamics of the unified field alone, the state of pure consciousness, pure awareness aware of itself."

If, however, we can speak of a "literature" of the Ved, doesn't that denote books and such? There are books known as the Vedas, which one can go to the library and read. If the Ved exists in consciousness, what are these books? How are they related to the Ved as the self-interacting dynamics of consciousness, and are they of any value to us in our desire to understand how natural law functions in the universe, particularly in the human body?

Describing the shruti aspect of the Ved, Maharishi explains that it refers to "those specific sounds that construct self-referral consciousness, which have been heard by the ancient seers in their own self-referral consciousness and are available to anyone at any time in one's own self-referral consciousness."

Maharishi traces the source of the Vedic tradition of knowledge all the way back to the dawn of creation, when great enlightened sages sat deep in meditation. Their awareness was so pure and refined that they heard the primordial sounds of natural law, the whisper of the unified field to itself, in their own consciousness. They directly experienced the self-interacting dynamics of consciousness within their own highly enlightened awareness. These sages passed this wisdom down orally from one generation to the next; much later on these primordial sounds were recorded and compiled by other great sages and teachers of the Vedic tradition. The Vedic literature is the record of these experiences of the enlightened.

Maharishi beautifully explains the connection of the Ved with human life. He says, "The knowledge of the unified field, Ved, is that self-whispering, self-interacting unified field which knows itself, which interacts with itself. We can very easily see this is the case of our own performance. There is some area within us from where thoughts and emotions arise, from where all behavior comes out. That is the area of the unified field within us; that is the Ved within us."

Thus, the Ved is not something separate from us, something to be studied in a library. The Ved is within us, it is the true nature of our own consciousness.

This underlines a major theme of this book: We want not only to understand the Ved intellectually; we want to know it on the level of direct experience as the self-interacting dynamics of our own consciousness. In fact, Maharishi's point is that this is the *only* way to really know the Ved.

If our nervous system is not refined enough to experience the self-referral dynamics of our own consciousness, then we cannot understand Vedic literature; we cannot comprehend the essentials of nature's creativity. There is nothing to be gained from reading the Vedic literature in the waking state of consciousness; we will only become confused by the descriptions of nature's mechanics, which are expressed from the reality of higher states of consciousness. If, however, our nervous system is refined enough to have the experience of pure consciousness, then on that basis, as we grow towards higher states of consciousness, eventually we can discover and know the same eternal laws of nature's creativity that were experienced and known to the ancient Vedic sages.

Knowledge gained in this manner is not in any way "borrowed" knowledge; it is created afresh through the experience of higher states of consciousness. When one has attained higher states of consciousness, it becomes valuable to read and study intellectually the Vedic texts, as a way to confirm the level of experience and knowledge gained in those states.

Maharishi comments on another common misconception about the Ved: "The word 'Ved' has been badly promoted to be a religion of some people in the Himalayas, out of sight and out of mind. Ved is a very, very good friend of us all. We say 'Ved' because that is the word by which it likes to be called—'Ved'. Ved is pure knowledge, and pure knowledge is organizing power."

Maharishi strongly emphasizes that the Ved is not confined to the people of one culture, nor is it a religion. Rather, it is a universal level of life that is the source of all knowledge in the universe, that is within each of us regardless of race or religion. It is our most intimate level of consciousness.

Here Maharishi also refers to another important principle of his Vedic Science, which he terms the organizing power of the Ved. He explains that the Ved has two main aspects: pure knowledge and its organizing power. The Ved itself is the field of pure knowledge. We know that any knowledge has value as knowledge; but it also has an applied value to achieve and accomplish, to create effects for oneself and in the world. In information theory, this principle is formulated in the principle that "knowledge has organizing power."

Maharishi explains that as the Ved represents the value of complete or pure knowledge, it therefore has the greatest organizing power—the infinite organizing power of nature. Here is Maharishi explaining this aspect of pure knowledge and its organizing power:

> Ved just means pure knowledge, and from information theory we know that knowledge has organizing power. Therefore, pure knowledge has pure organizing power—total, infinite organizing power. This is a very clear intellectual perception of the infinite organizing power lying within us.
>
> The knowledge of the Ved declares that this totality of knowledge and infinite organizing power is myself; it is thyself; it is this, that, and everything. The total potential of natural law is lively within ourselves. It is guiding our activity, and it is responsible for all the world that we have. The unified field, speaking to itself, interacting with itself, is nothing other than our own Self.

Maharishi also points out that when we experience this field, this total infinite organizing power of natural law becomes lively within our own awareness: "Human awareness opening itself to this beautiful field of all possibilities becomes lively in the field of all possibilities."

The recognition of the inherent organizing power of natural law within us is beautifully illustrated in modern physiology. The DNA molecule contained in virtually every cell of the body exists as a source of pure information. This information simultaneously contains the organizing power to create and regulate all the complex forms and functions of our human body.

The basis of the knowledge and organizing power of DNA is, of course, ultimately the Ved, the primordial sounds of the self-interacting dynamics of pure consciousness. These are found expressed in the Rik Ved, Sam Ved, Yajur Ved, and Atharv Ved.

Vedic Literature: The Sequential Unfoldment of Natural Law from the Self to the Universe

Several times I have referred to the principle in Maharishi's Vedic Science that the structure of Vedic literature expresses the structure of the universe. Maharishi explains that in this structure, it is the *sequence* of Vedic literature that is important: the unfoldment of the Vedic literature exactly expresses the sequential unfoldment of natural law from its unified state in pure transcendental consciousness to its expressions in the whole universe. "The structure of pure knowledge itself is so sequentially organized," Maharishi explains, "that its sequence resembles the sequential growth of natural law from the unmanifest to the finer fields of the manifest world to the whole universe. The sequence is important."

In the following passage, Maharishi reviews the order of the various sections of Vedic literature, again emphasizing how its "perfect sequence" expresses the orderly unfoldment of natural law in the human body and in the universe.

> Perfect precision and order in perfect sequence is available in the arrangement of the Vedic literature: the Samhitas, the Upanishads, the Brahmanas, and Aranyakas; the Shiksha, Kalp, Vyakaran, Nirukt, Chhandas, and Jyotish; the Nyaya, Vaisheshik, Sankhya, Yog, Karm Mimans, and Vedant; the Smritis, Itihas, and Puranas; and the Upa-Ved—Ayur-Ved, Gandharv Ved, Dhanur-Ved, and Sthapatya Ved. These are the different aspects of the Vedic literature, which, organized in this sequence, give us the sequential progression of the whole

body and behavior and the whole universal creation—all well regu-
lated in the evolutionary direction.

The following is a list of the Vedic literature, expressing the
sequential unfoldment of natural law "from the unmanifest to the finer
fields of the manifest world to the whole universe":

Samhitas	Rik Ved		**Upangas**	Nyaya
	Sam Ved			Vaisheshika
	Yajur-Ved			Sankhya
	Atharv Ved			Yog
Brahmanas	Upanishads			Karm Mimans
	Aranyakas			Vedant
	Brahmanas		**Itihas**	
Vedangas	Shiksha		**Puran**	
	Kalp		**Smriti**	
	Vyakaran		**Upa-Ved**	Ayur-Ved
	Nirukt			Gandharv Ved
	Chhandas			Dhanur-Ved
	Jyotish			Sthapatya Ved

The Vedic literature elaborates different, specific values of Rishi, Devata, and Chhandas

In his Vedic Science, Maharishi has provided a unique and complete
approach to intellectually understanding the Ved. Maharishi explains
that the entire Vedic literature is like a tree with many limbs and
branches. The transformations of Rishi, Devata, and Chhandas into
one another, arising from the eternal self-interacting dynamics of the
Samhita—the reverberations of fully awake consciousness within
itself—are displayed in their totality in the Rik Ved, and are elaborated
in the various branches of the Vedic literature. Each of the different
modes of consciousness—Samhita of Rishi, Devata, and Chhandas—
has a very specific technical meaning. We have already understood
Samhita as the unbounded wholeness of consciousness, fully awake
within itself;* and Rishi, Devata, and Chhandas as the knower,
processes of knowing, and the known (Maharishi sometimes also
describes them as "observer, process of observation, and observed"). In
addition, Maharishi explains that Rishi is the witnessing quality within

the wakeful quality of Samhita; Devata is the transformational quality of consciousness, the value of activity or dynamism; and Chhandas is the structural quality of consciousness, also defined as "that which hides"—the concrete, structural value which obscures the wakeful quality of consciousness within. Each section of the Vedic literature can thus be understood as expressing primarily either the Rishi, Devata, or Chhandas aspect of natural law.

How the primordial sounds of the Ved sequentially unfold

Maharishi's Vedic Science includes a step-by-step analysis of the mechanics through which all the sounds and syllables of the Vedic literature unfold.

Maharishi's analysis begins with the very first sounds of the Vedic literature and the process of self-interaction by which they emerge. It then traces the elaboration of the primordial sounds of the Ved through all the following verses and collections of verses. With this approach it is possible to trace the unfoldment of the diverse branches of the Vedic literature from the self-interaction of the Samhita of Rishi, Devata, and Chhandas.

In Chapter 2 we discussed Maharishi's explanation of how the *intelligence* value of consciousness discriminates the three diverse values of Rishi, Devata, and Chhandas within its unified state (Samhita). In Maharishi's words,

> The unbounded sea of intelligence quietly scans its own structure, and, maintaining its unified status, spontaneously recognizes its own nature to be a combination of three values—the observer, the process of observation, and the observed; . . . and all the three together in their unified state—one singularity of pure intelligence, analyzing itself into three qualities, maintains them eternally in its unified state—Samhita of Rishi, Devata, and Chhandas.

---

* From this discussion, it may be apparent that there are two shades of meaning in Maharishi's explanation of Samhita. We are already familiar with Samhita as the unity value or unified state of Rishi, Devata, and Chhandas. Maharishi also refers to the Samhita of the Ved, or the Samhitas—meaning the four principal Vedas: Rik, Sam, Yajur, and Atharv. Both meanings refer to the pure knowledge aspect of the Ved, the laws of nature as they unfold within pure consciousness through the self-interacting dynamics of consciousness. In Maharishi's words, "The Samhita is the structure of total natural law. Samhita is the basic aspect of Vedic literature, the Ved as such, the structure of pure knowledge."

It is the interaction of what Maharishi terms the different "intellectually conceived components of this unified, self-referral state of consciousness" which constitutes "that all-powerful activity at the most elementary level of nature. . . . , [which] is responsible for the innumerable varieties of life in the world, the innumerable streams of intelligence in creation."

This value of intelligence, Maharishi explains, which is awake to the three diversified values of Rishi, Devata, and Chhandas within its own unified state, is the basis of all the different expanding modes of intelligence sequentially expressed in the Vedic literature.

Let's follow Maharishi's analysis of this very refined level of nature's functioning. Maharishi's insight is expressed in the Vedic expression from the Yog Sutras: *Vritti sarupyam itaratra*—"What you see, you become." This is the principle governing the self-interaction of Rishi, Devata, Chhandas, and Samhita.

The Samhita value of pure consciousness, fully awake within itself, is perpetually aware of its fundamental constituents—Rishi, Devata, and Chhandas—within its unified structure. Because all are modes of pure consciousness, each is awake to all of the other values. Rishi is awake to itself and to everything else; Devata is awake to itself and everything else, and so on.

The Samhita, in its awareness of Rishi, Devata, and Chhandas, spontaneously unfolds with the awareness of each one. That is, it begins to play the role of each of these three values. In this process the Samhita value becomes transformed; this is how transformations are created within pure consciousness.

Maharishi explains that the Rik Ved expresses the Samhita value of consciousness—the totality of natural law. When the Rishi value of intelligence "sees itself"—is awake to itself—in terms of the Samhita (another way to say this is that Rik Ved or Rik Samhita is seen from the perspective of Rishi), the Samhita becomes transformed. This transformation is responsible for the sounds of Sam Ved. When the Devata value of intelligence sees itself in terms of Samhita it becomes transformed, and thus Yajur Ved is produced. And likewise, when Chhandas views itself in terms of Samhita, the sounds of Atharv Ved are produced. Thus, Sam Ved expresses primarily the Rishi value of intelligence, Yajur Ved the Devata value, and Atharv Ved the Chhandas value. Maharishi describes this aspect of the Vedic literature:

> The whole Vedic literature is dedicated to bringing out these three values in terms of Rishi, Devata, and Chhandas. There is one Ved, called Rik Ved, which is the totality of all knowledge. Knowledge means knowledge of the three. There are three Vedas basically attributed to the three values of Rishi, Devata, and Chhandas. They are Sam Ved, Yajur Ved, and Atharv Ved.

As Rishi, Devata, and Chhandas view themselves with respect to the Samhita and each other, this continuing self-interaction gives rise to still other transformations. Maharishi goes on to explain that the next sections that arise in the sequential unfoldment of Vedic literature—the Upanishads, Aranyakas, and Brahmanas (all three are known collectively as the Brahmanas)—display these further permutations: "These three values of Rishi, Devata, and Chhandas have been expounded as three distinct values by three aspects of the Vedic literature: Upanishads, Aranyakas, and Brahmanas." The Brahmanas as a whole display what Maharishi terms the infinite organizing power of pure knowledge; they bring out further values of intelligence found in the Samhita.

The intelligence aspect of pure consciousness continues to discriminate, creating innumerable permutations of Rishi, Devata, Chhandas, and Samhita. Each subsequent area of the Vedic literature—the six Vedangas, the six Upangas, and the Itihas, Puran, Smriti, and Upa-Ved—is a further elaboration of these fundamental transformations of consciousness. The process of unfoldment through these sequential transformations is known as Maharishi's *Veda Lila* ("the play of the Ved"). Eventually all possible transformations are exhausted and the fullness of infinite diversity of the universe emerges.

The transition from consciousness to matter
in the sequential unfoldment of natural law

The sequence of the various sections of the Vedic literature follows the progression of the laws of nature—from the purely abstract level of the self-interacting dynamics within pure consciousness—to the point at which they begin to manifest in concrete form as matter—to their full expression as all the forms and phenomena in the universe.

I referred earlier to the principle in Maharishi's Vedic Science of *nam rup*, name and form: as the laws of nature are expressed as primordial sounds, the form of each aspect of natural law is inherent in the sound itself. The concrete material form is simply the more precipitated expression of that particular vibratory quality of sound.

Maharishi explains this process in detail, describing the "impulses of intelligence expressed as *shruti* (sounds) of the self-interacting dynamics of consciousness, which, fully awake in its organizing power, is the administering intelligence of the universe." He explains how consciousness is expressed in primordial sound, which continues to expand and becomes the Rik Ved: "In the process of manifestation of sounds, the self-interacting dynamics of consciousness, administering itself . . . manifests as primordial sound and continues to expand into the structure of Rik Ved."

Maharishi describes how, as the process of evolution of creation from consciousness to matter continues, the unmanifest frequencies of sounds become audible frequencies, and the *tanmatras* are created. (In Chapter 5, we discussed the tanmatras as the finest level of matter in creation, on the "borderline" between consciousness and the body, which are associated with the five senses.) From the tanmatras then arise the material particles which become the organs and systems of the body, and the physical universe:

> Continuance of the process of evolution of consciousness transforms the self-referral frequencies of the primordial sound (unmanifest) into audible frequencies of sound, and these frequencies (tanmatras), in their process of evolution, create material particles giving rise to the auditory system (sense of hearing, etc.)

Thus, we can see from Maharishi's analysis that in the unfoldment of the Vedic literature, the further sections represent the concrete, more precipitated material expressions of the values of consciousness found in the Samhita of Rik Ved. The intelligence of nature continues to expand, creating as it goes all the values of the expanding, diversifying universe, and this is reflected in the structure of the Vedic literature.

While the complete body of Vedic literature is vast and complex, its different parts can be understood in terms of Maharishi's insight into their expression of different values of Rishi, Devata, and Chhandas found in the Samhita of the Ved. The diagram on the following page

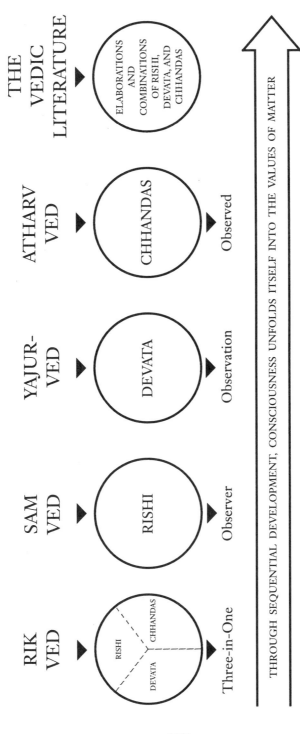

Ved—The Script of Nature

RIK VED	SAM VED	YAJUR-VED	ATHARV VED	THE VEDIC LITERATURE
Three-in-One	Observer	Observation	Observed	

RISHI · CHHANDAS · DEVATA

RISHI · DEVATA · CHHANDAS · ELABORATIONS AND COMBINATIONS OF RISHI, DEVATA, AND CHHANDAS

THROUGH SEQUENTIAL DEVELOPMENT, CONSCIOUSNESS UNFOLDS ITSELF INTO THE VALUES OF MATTER

Ved is a clear script of the self-referral state of pure consciousness, the togetherness of observer (Rishi), observation (Devata), and observed (Chhandas). • The whole of Vedic literature is dedicated to bringing out the details of the three-in-one structure of pure knowledge. Rik Ved is the totality of all knowledge—the knowledge of the three-in-one. Sam Ved is basically attributed to the value of Rishi, Yajur-Ved to Devata, and Atharv Ved to Chhandas. All the other aspects of Vedic literature expound these three values, detailing the perpetually self-referral transformation through the steps of sequential development by which consciousness, the Self, gets into the value of matter, the body.

expresses this general principle governing how the Vedic literature unfolds through the sequential elaborations of the Samhita of Rishi, Devata, and Chhandas.

The Entire Universe is Administered by Consciousness

Maharishi has brought to light many more rich permutations of the process of unfoldment of the Ved, which can be seen in the interrelationships of the various branches of the Vedic literature. Our explanation here has given us just a taste of the gems of knowledge to be found in the deeply fulfilling and enlightening field of Vedic study.

The great significance of this knowledge for us is in understanding how the universe described in the Ved is administered from our own self-referral consciousness. Maharishi has recently been emphasizing the theme of perfect administration for individuals and governments, through enlivening the self-referral quality of consciousness that administers human life and the entire universe. As he explains,

> All fields of creation are the diverse projections of self-referral consciousness, and, as they always maintain connectedness with their source, the entire field of diversity is the field of consciousness. That is why self-referral consciousness administering itself means the entire universe is administered by consciousness.

In describing this phenomenon, Maharishi emphasizes that it is based on the simultaneous coexistence of unity and diversity within pure consciousness. All the diversity in the universe is held together by its connection to the field of unity, or "togetherness," at its source in the Samhita.

The diagram on the next page shows once again the relationship of the Samhita and Rishi, Devata, and Chhandas, this time illustrating that all activity in the universe is "administered" from the level of unity or "togetherness" in the Samhita of Rik Ved. Maharishi comments:

> The reins of the diversifying universe are being held by the unifying quality at its basis.
>
> It is enlightening to see the diversifying phenomenon of the ever-evolving Rishi, Devata, and Chhandas being held at their source, Samhita.
>
> It is enlightening to see the structure of pure intelligence in two qualities lively within the self-referral state of consciousness: (1) unity

and (2) diversity, simultaneously—unity of its own self-referral state of pure wakefulness, and diversity of the three qualities that constitute the self-referral dynamics of unity—observer, process of observing, and observed.

It is the Samhita quality of consciousness that holds the reins of all activity in the universe; Samhita, the fully self-referral consciousness, administers the universe.

And what is the field of pure, self-referral consciousness? It is our own Self.

Through Maharishi's insight we can understand how the vast array of elements in the physical universe, from DNA to the galaxies, are expressions of the fundamental dynamics of natural law in the field of pure consciousness—what Maharishi terms "the government of nature." As Maharishi beautifully explains,

> It is the same silent functioning of the government of nature that transforms the earth into diamond and gold; it is the same silent functioning of the government of nature that produces a tree from an empty seed; it is the same government of nature that transforms mud into the beautiful lotus, colorless sap into the beautiful, tender, pink petal; it is the same government of nature that maintains the orderly

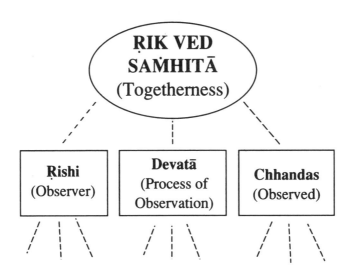

growth of life and harmony in the infinite dynamism of the galactic universe; it is the same government of nature that renders consciousness, a non-physical reality, to appear as a physical reality.

The absolute creative intelligence (the government of nature) eternally established in its self-referral state, fully alert and awake, most spontaneously, most innocently administers the universe, and spontaneously, most naturally, from within everything and everyone, maintains the destiny of everything and everyone.

All this knowledge is contained in the Vedic literature, which thus contains the knowledge of every area of subjective and objective life, and of how to bring it to perfection. Thus, Maharishi's Vedic Science shows us the connection between the Ved, the universe, and our own life.

Pure Knowledge and Its Infinite Organizing Power

I want to comment a little further on just a few specific aspects of the Vedic literature that are of practical interest to us as we explore the applied value of Maharishi's Vedic Science for physiology and health.

Maharishi explains that the two major aspects of the Ved we have referred to earlier—pure knowledge and its organizing power—are expressed by the *mantra* aspect of the Ved and the *Brahman* aspect of the Ved. As we discussed earlier, the mantras or sounds of the four principal Vedas express pure knowledge, and the Brahmanas contain the organizing power of the mantra aspect of the Ved. Maharishi further explains that the Brahmanas are the applied aspect of the Ved, which he also refers to as Vedic technology.

Thus the "technology" in Maharishi's Vedic Science and Technology refers to specific, skillful uses of the sound value, the mantras, of the Ved to create, from the level of the self-interacting dynamics of consciousness, transformations on the outer, expressed level of life, including the concrete level of matter. Maharishi refers this to as Vedic engineering. The specific technologies used in Vedic engineering are the yagyas, which we mentioned in Chapter 6, the knowledge of which is contained in the Brahmanas.

The knowledge of the TM-Sidhi program is contained in the Yog Sutras of Patanjali, one of the six Upangas. Thus the Vedic literature contains the ultimate self-referral knowledge for human life: the Ved contains the knowledge of how to experience its own self-interacting dynamics, and thereby allow the human mind, body, and behavior to develop to enlightenment.

Role of Ayur-Ved in the Sequential Unfoldment of Natural Law

The Upa-Ved is also of special interest to us. Maharishi explains that as the stream of evolution in the unfoldment of natural law continues, the Upa-Ved arises at the point where the end of the transformations within consciousness has been reached, and consciousness has assumed the quality of matter: "In the sequential growth, consciousness becomes matter. Then what we find is that the field of Ved as consciousness is over and the field of Ayur-Ved has come up to deal with matter."

Ayur-Ved is one of the four branches of the Upa-Ved, or "subordinate Ved," which presents the knowledge of how to enliven the Ved as a living reality on the level of one's own existence. The Upa-Ved provides the principles and techniques through which matter can be re-enlivened with the full value of consciousness. We can now more fully appreciate the significance of all the techniques and approaches of Maharishi Ayur-Ved we discussed earlier in the book (Gandharv Ved is also part of the Upa-Ved), in light of their value in "re-enlivening the full value of consciousness in the field of matter (the body)."

Earlier we discussed the three doshas, vat, pitt, and kaph, the governing principles in the body. Now we can better understand their emergence in the sequential unfoldment of the Ved as the finest material expressions of the principles of consciousness, Rishi, Devata, and Chhandas.

We also understood earlier the goal of Maharishi Ayur-Ved to create balance among vat, pitt, and kaph. We can now understand this as a further elaboration of the commentary of the Ved upon itself: as natural law sequentially unfolds, vat, pitt, and kaph emerge as the further expressions of consciousness—of Rishi, Devata, and Chhandas—in the field of matter. The way to maintain balance among vat, pitt, and kaph is thus to maintain their self-referral connection with their unified source in the Samhita of pure consciousness. This is the purpose of all the approaches and treatments of Maharishi Ayur-Ved.

As 1993 was just beginning, Maharishi commented on the curriculum of the College of Maharishi Ayur-Ved, founded the previous year at MIU. He emphasized the importance of students' mastering

Ayurvedic pulse diagnosis as a means of attending to the finest level of intelligence in the body, correcting imbalances and creating balance from that level. Describing this "approach through intelligence," he referred to a *sloca* (verse) from Charak Samhita, one of the classical texts of Ayur-Ved in the Vedic literature:

> "*Purusham, purusham vrich. . . .*" This means, "Look to the intelligence at the grain level of physiology; the intelligence which witnesses every grain of physiology." That witnessing intelligence must be lively in every grain of physiology—otherwise, there will be some imbalance on the level of performance of prakriti [nature]. It will be like a millionaire descending to the level of his accountant; so we must attend to the witnessing intelligence in every grain. This is the approach through intelligence, to correct all imbalance. In this, the pulse will tell us how much the physiology is self-referral, and how much it has gone out of the self-referral state.

Maharishi went on to explain that the aim of pulse diagnosis is to fathom the level of the most fundamental mechanics of natural law in the patient's physiology—the point "where Rishi, Devata, and Chhandas emerge from the Samhita" and from which the whole Vedic literature emerges:

> We feel in the pulse different levels, different layers. For example, we can feel the Vedang, Upang, and Upa-Ved levels in the pulse. The whole Vedic literature emerges from the point where Rishi, Devata, and Chhandas emerge from Samhita. The aim in pulse diagnosis is to feel at this point.

From Maharishi's explanation it is evident that the whole Vedic literature is lively in the physiology of every human being. Thus, when the Ayurvedic physician has developed the ability to feel the pulse at these levels of the physiology corresponding to the Vedangas, Upangas, etc., then he or she can locate where any imbalance has arisen.

This principle is at the foundation of the purpose and goal of Maharishi Ayur-Ved, to enliven the self-referral field of pure knowledge at the basis of the physiology, and on that basis to create balance in the field of the expression of knowledge, the body. As Maharishi explains,

> Ayur-Ved deals with the totality of life from the field of matter. It also prescribes the approach to regaining balance from the field of con-

sciousness. It attends to the totality of the field of knowledge and to the field of the expression of knowledge, matter. Ayur-Ved deals with consciousness and matter. Working from both points of view, it recreates a very balanced personality. This is the approach of Ayur-Ved.

The knowledge of the Ved, Maharishi explains, handles the entire field of science and technology in terms of oneself. It covers infinite diversity and eternal unity and puts them together in one package of knowledge. Fortunate for us, the students of Maharishi's Vedic Science, and for all of humanity, is the rise in this generation of this enormously complete range of knowledge, encompassing its applied value that includes practical technologies of Maharishi Ayur-Ved and the other branches of the Vedic literature to bring solutions to the problems of humanity.

Most fortunate of all, we can have this very complete knowledge in the simplest form of human awareness, which is also, we must not forget, a field of total bliss consciousness—the level, in Maharishi's words, "where Heaven reigns, harmony, happiness, peace reigns." Because of this, Maharishi points out, we can create from the self-referral field of bliss in our own consciousness waves of bliss in our physiology. And this, he explains, is the basis on which we can create not only bliss throughout our lives, but Heaven on Earth.

14

RIK VED: THE CONSTITUTION
OF THE UNIVERSE

ULL-PAGE ANNOUNCEMENTS OF THE CONSTITUTION OF the Universe appeared in January 1992, in newspapers and magazines throughout the world. The announcements were headlined: "Maharishi invites all governments to create Heaven on Earth in their countries by bringing their national constitutions into alliance with the Constitution of the Universe and thereby raising governmental administration to be as efficient and as effective as the Government of Nature."

The main body of the ad featured an elaborate graphic display of the Sanskrit syllables in the first sukt of Rik Ved. Below this was an equally elaborate graphic of the mathematical symbols used to describe the "Lagrangian" of superstring theory—the latest and most successful unified quantum field theory, widely seen as uniting all the fundamental forces in nature. These graphics appear on pages 236–237.

When Maharishi made this great discovery of the Constitution of the Universe, as we saw in Chapter 2, he predicted that the sequential structure of sounds in the Ved would have its exact correspondence in the mathematical formulas of the most advanced areas of physics. He worked closely with MIU's Dr. John Hagelin, a world authority in unified quantum field theories, to bring out the detailed and precise set of parallels between the sequential structure of Maharishi's cognition of Rik Ved, and the description of natural law found in the most compact expressions of Superstring theory. The results of Dr. Hagelin's research are shown in the chart of the Lagrangian of the superstring. The Lagrangian is the most detailed mathematical expression of the structure and dynamics of the unified field of natural law.

This precise mathematical correspondence between the descriptions of the detailed structure of natural law provided by modern science and by Maharishi's Vedic Science—both on the verbal level of nature's language, and on the mathematical level of symbols—reveal that these two descriptions of the most fundamental level of natural law, the Constitution of the Universe, are identical. It also shows that these two great traditions of knowledge, objective and subjective—modern and ancient—uphold one another in providing what Maharishi terms "the timely knowledge of natural law which alone is competent to eliminate problems and to raise the quality of life in society to the level of Heaven on Earth."

"The clear and electric implication of this equivalence," explains Dr. Hagelin, "is that human beings can experience—and harness—the concentrated source of orderliness at the unified basis of nature's functioning." Dr. Hagelin presented this knowledge to over 2,600 physicists in the past year, in a tour of 20 European universities and research institutions.

To grasp more fully the significance of the Constitution of the Universe, and why Maharishi considers it of such vital importance to the future of the world, we must probe more deeply into the structure of Rik Ved as brought to light by Maharishi.

Maharishi's Apaurusheya Bhashya of the Ved

One of Maharishi's most important contributions to the revival of Vedic Science is his Apaurusheya Bhashya. As we explained earlier, the word apaurusheya means "uncreated"—that is, not created by human minds, but a spontaneous expression of the laws of nature. Maharishi's Apaurusheya Bhashya is therefore the "uncreated commentary" of the Ved. It reveals the inherent perfection of the structure of the Ved, by which the Samhita provides its own commentary.

This commentary of the Ved upon itself is found in the various

The Constitution

These figures display the main sections of the chart of the Constitution of the Universe, which bring out the precise set of parallels between the descriptions of the detailed structure of natural law provided by modern science and by Maharishi's Vedic Science. The three upper boxes display, from the standpoint of Maharishi's Vedic Science, the self-interacting dynamics in the structure of Rik Ved Samhita as brought to light by Maharishi's Apaurusheya Bhashya of the Ved. The three lower boxes depict precisely the same mathematical structure of sequential unfoldment of natural law in the Lagrangian of the superstring, which represents the most complete mathematical expression of the unified field of natural law.

Ahamkar	Buddhi	Manas	Akash	Vayu	Agni	Jal	Prithivi
अक्	नि	मी	ळे	पु	रो	हि	तं
AK	NI	MI	LE	PU	RO	HI	TAM
सु	मिः	पु	वे	षि	अं	षि	धि
सु	मि	नां	उ	यि	मं	रन	वु
व	गे	यं	यु	ञ	मं	ख्व	रं
सु	मि	हो	तां	रा	कि	कं	तुः
य	ड	ऋ	दा	शु	षे	तु	वं
उ	पं	त्वा	ये	दि	वे	दिं	वे
रा	जं	नत	म	ख्व	रा	षीं	गो
स	नः	षिु	ते	वं	सु	न	वे

$$\underset{\substack{\text{D=10 Heterotic}\\\text{Superstring}}}{} \mathcal{L}_F^{(10)} = \frac{1}{\pi}\left(\psi_1^i\partial_-\psi_1^i + \psi_2^i\partial_-\psi_2^i + \psi_3^i\partial_-\psi_3^i + \psi_4^i\partial_-\psi_4^i + \psi_5^i\partial_-\psi_5^i + \psi_6^i\partial_-\psi_6^i + \psi_7^i\partial_-\psi_7^i + \psi_8^i\partial_-\psi_8^i\right)$$

$$\underset{\substack{\text{D=4 Heterotic}\\\text{Superstring}}}{} \mathcal{L}_F^{(4)} = \frac{1}{\pi}\big(\overline{\psi}_1^i\partial_-\overline{\psi}_1^i + \overline{\psi}_2^i\partial_-\overline{\psi}_2^i + \chi_L^1\partial_-\chi_L^1 + \chi_L^2\partial_-\chi_L^2 + \chi_L^3\partial_-\chi_L^3 + \chi_L^4\partial_-\chi_L^4 + \chi_L^5\partial_-\chi_L^5 + \chi_L^6\partial_-\chi_L^6$$
$$+ y_L^1\partial_-y_L^1 + y_L^2\partial_-y_L^2 + y_L^3\partial_-y_L^3 + y_L^4\partial_-y_L^4 + y_L^5\partial_-y_L^5 + y_L^6\partial_-y_L^6 + \omega_L^1\partial_-\omega_L^1 + \omega_L^2\partial_-\omega_L^2$$
$$+ \omega_L^3\partial_-\omega_L^3 + \omega_L^4\partial_-\omega_L^4 + \omega_L^5\partial_-\omega_L^5 + \omega_L^6\partial_-\omega_L^6 + \overline{y}_R^1\partial_-\overline{y}_R^1 + \overline{y}_R^2\partial_-\overline{y}_R^2 + \overline{y}_R^3\partial_-\overline{y}_R^3 + \overline{y}_R^4\partial_-\overline{y}_R^4$$
$$+ \overline{y}_R^5\partial_-\overline{y}_R^5 + \overline{y}_R^6\partial_-\overline{y}_R^6 + \overline{\omega}_R^1\partial_-\overline{\omega}_R^1 + \overline{\omega}_R^2\partial_-\overline{\omega}_R^2 + \overline{\omega}_R^3\partial_-\overline{\omega}_R^3 + \overline{\omega}_R^4\partial_-\overline{\omega}_R^4 + \overline{\omega}_R^5\partial_-\overline{\omega}_R^5 + \overline{\omega}_R^6\partial_-\overline{\omega}_R^6$$
$$+ \psi_R^1\partial_-\psi_R^1 + \psi_R^2\partial_-\psi_R^2 + \psi_R^3\partial_-\psi_R^3 + \psi_R^4\partial_-\psi_R^4 + \psi_R^5\partial_-\psi_R^5 + \eta_R^1\partial_-\eta_R^1 + \eta_R^2\partial_-\eta_R^2 + \eta_R^3\partial_-\eta_R^3$$
$$+ \overline{\psi}_R^1\partial_-\overline{\psi}_R^1 + \overline{\psi}_R^2\partial_-\overline{\psi}_R^2 + \overline{\psi}_R^3\partial_-\overline{\psi}_R^3 + \overline{\psi}_R^4\partial_-\overline{\psi}_R^4 + \overline{\psi}_R^5\partial_-\overline{\psi}_R^5 + \overline{\eta}_R^1\partial_-\overline{\eta}_R^1 + \overline{\eta}_R^2\partial_-\overline{\eta}_R^2 + \overline{\eta}_R^3\partial_-\overline{\eta}_R^3$$
$$+ \phi_R^1\partial_-\phi_R^1 + \phi_R^2\partial_-\phi_R^2 + \phi_R^3\partial_-\phi_R^3 + \phi_R^4\partial_-\phi_R^4 + \phi_R^5\partial_-\phi_R^5 + \phi_R^6\partial_-\phi_R^6 + \phi_R^7\partial_-\phi_R^7 + \phi_R^8\partial_-\phi_R^8$$
$$+ \overline{\phi}_R^1\partial_-\overline{\phi}_R^1 + \overline{\phi}_R^2\partial_-\overline{\phi}_R^2 + \overline{\phi}_R^3\partial_-\overline{\phi}_R^3 + \overline{\phi}_R^4\partial_-\overline{\phi}_R^4 + \overline{\phi}_R^5\partial_-\overline{\phi}_R^5 + \overline{\phi}_R^6\partial_-\overline{\phi}_R^6 + \overline{\phi}_R^7\partial_-\overline{\phi}_R^7 + \overline{\phi}_R^8\partial_-\overline{\phi}_R^8\big)$$

stages of the sequential unfoldment of the Vedic literature. Maharishi's Apaurusheya Bhashya explains how the Ved spontaneously and sequentially unfolds from the most compactified possible form of pure knowledge. This is analogous to a seed, which contains in a concentrated form the potential for the entire tree. The seed contains all the knowledge the tree will need for the sequential growth of its trunk, branches, leaves, fruits, and flowers. The parts of the tree can be said to unfold as "commentary" on the knowledge contained in the seed.

The full unfoldment of pure knowledge is displayed in its most elaborated form as all the different branches of the Vedic literature. This is the full-grown tree of knowledge. The same knowledge can be seen in more compact form at different stages in its sequential unfoldment. For example, Maharishi has explained that the complete knowledge of every branch of the Vedic literature—the Vedang, Upang, Itihas, Puran, and Smriti—can be located in the Samhitas, the four principal Vedas (Rik, Sam, Yajur, Atharv), in a highly concentrated form.

The totality of knowledge is contained more compactly in the Rik Ved itself. It is found in a still more concentrated form in the first collection of verses of Rik Ved, referred to in Sanskrit as the first *mandal*,

of the Universe

Ahamkar	Buddhi	Manas	Akash	Vayu	Agni	Jal	Prithivi
यु	ज्ञ	स्यें	दे	व	मृ	त्वि	जंम्
YA	JNA	SYA	DE	VA	MRI	TVI	JAM
रों	ड	घों	नुं	तं	नै	हुं	त
त्यों	यं	में	ब	दिं	वे	दिं	वे
वि	ध्व	तः	प	रिं	भु	र	सिं
सु	त्यं	शिचुं	ॠ	श्रं	ब	स्त	मः
ब्य	मैं	घ्रं	इं	क	रि	घ्य	सिं
दो	षां	ब	स्त	र्घि	या	बु	·यम्
पा	मृं	तं	स्यं	दी	दिं	वि	म्
ब्य	मैं	सूं	पा	यं	नों	भं	ब

Ahamkar	Buddhi	Manas	Akash	Vayu	Agni	Jal	Prithivi
हों	तां	रं	र	त्लुं	धा	तं	मम्
स	दें	वां	ए	ह	ब	च	ति
यु	श	सं	व्रीं	र	ब	त	मम्
दें	इ	हें	बे	यूं	भि	ग	च्छं
त	बे	त	त्सुं	त्यं	मं	झुं	रः
न	मों	भ	रं	त्लुं	ए	में	सि
व	धैं	मा	जं	सुं	बे	द	में
स	च	सुं	आं	नः	स्खु	स्त	दे

$$\mathcal{L}_F^{(10)} = \frac{1}{\pi}(\psi^1_L\partial_r\psi^1_L + \psi^2_L\partial_r\psi^2_L + \psi^3_L\partial_r\psi^3_L + \psi^4_L\partial_r\psi^4_L + \psi^5_L\partial_r\psi^5_L + \psi^6_L\partial_r\psi^6_L + \psi^7_L\partial_r\psi^7_L + \psi^8_L\partial_r\psi^8_L$$

$$\mathcal{L}_F^{(4)} = \frac{1}{\pi}(\overline{\psi}^1_L\partial_r\overline{\psi}^1_L + \overline{\psi}^2_L\partial_r\overline{\psi}^2_L + \chi^1_L\partial_r\chi^1_L + \chi^2_L\partial_r\chi^2_L + \chi^3_L\partial_r\chi^3_L + \chi^4_L\partial_r\chi^4_L + \chi^5_L\partial_r\chi^5_L + \chi^6_L\partial_r\chi^6_L$$

$$\mathcal{L}_F^{(10)} = \frac{1}{\pi}(\psi^1_L\partial_r\psi^1_L + \psi^2_L\partial_r\psi^2_L + \psi^3_L\partial_r\psi^3_L + \psi^4_L\partial_r\psi^4_L + \psi^5_L\partial_r\psi^5_L + \psi^6_L\partial_r\psi^6_L + \psi^7_L\partial_r\psi^7_L + \psi^8_L\partial_r\psi^8_L$$

$$\mathcal{L}_F^{(4)} = \frac{1}{\pi}(\overline{\psi}^1_L\partial_r\overline{\psi}^1_L + \overline{\psi}^2_L\partial_r\overline{\psi}^2_L + \chi^1_L\partial_r\chi^1_L + \chi^2_L\partial_r\chi^2_L + \chi^3_L\partial_r\chi^3_L + \chi^4_L\partial_r\chi^4_L + \chi^5_L\partial_r\chi^5_L + \chi^6_L\partial_r\chi^6_L$$

and in an even more concentrated form in the first *sukt* (stanza). It is found in a yet more concentrated form in the first *richa* (verse) of Rik Ved—the first 24 syllables of the first sukt. This complete knowledge is again contained in the first *pad*, or first eight syllables of the first rich; and finally, it is found in its most concentrated form in the first syllable of the Ved: 'AK'.

This explains how the Ved can be said to contain its own commentary. Its structure is like a set of nested boxes, one within the other. Each box contains the whole, yet each larger one is a more elaborate version of the smaller ones. This process whereby a very concentrated seed of knowledge manifests sequentially into more and more elaborate and expressed forms is universal throughout nature. It is vividly illustrated in biological phenomena, where one single fertilized cell gives rise to an enormously complex organism. The entire process by which organisms unfold from one cell to very complex tissues, organs, and integrated physiological systems is completely natural and spontaneous. Each part, each cell, contains in its DNA the entire knowledge governing its complete development, and each stage of development arrives as the further elaboration or display of that knowledge contained in the DNA.

The unique insight of Maharishi's Apaurusheya Bhashya is how these sequential and spontaneous mechanics of development in the Ved unfold through the dynamics of consciousness. One important aspect of the Apaurusheya Bhashya is an understanding of the gaps.

Gaps of Silence

Maharishi has explained that in the sequential progression of the primordial sounds of the Ved are gaps of silence. For example, the first syllable of Rik Ved is AK. The transition from 'A' to 'K' involves the collapse of the sound A and the emergence of the next sound, K. Thus there is a gap between A and K, and this gap and all the other gaps between syllables throughout Rik Ved play an extremely important role. They have fundamental significance in this entire process of spontaneous, sequential unfoldment, because each gap contains the complete dynamics of natural law—the mechanics of transformation—responsible for the emergence of creation. Thus, not only is the *sequence* of the various sections of the Vedic literature important for understanding the total mechanics of creation. As we will see, it is in the sequential progression of sound and *silence* that the true meaning and content of the Ved reside (not on the level of intellectual meanings ascribed to the Ved in various translations).

Maharishi explains that each succeeding expression of sound arises from the specific mechanics of transformation present in the gap that precedes it. These mechanics of transformation involve four distinct stages.

The first stage involves the collapse of the first sound. This is referred to in Sanskrit as *pradhvansabhav*. The second stage, *atyantabhav*, is the state of non-activity, involving the total annihilation of the syllable to the unmanifest silence of pure consciousness. The third stage, *anyonyabhav*, is a state of all possibilities. In pure consciousness exist all the lively transformations or self-interacting dynamics of consciousness. These self-interacting dynamics structure the fourth and final stage, *pragabhav*, the emergence of the next syllable. Thus in every gap is the unmanifest dynamism of silence which ensures the orderly unfoldment of knowledge.

Maharishi uses an analogy to describe this process of transformation. When a swimmer dives into the waters of the Caribbean, he dives at one point with a particular angle. This is like the first stage of the gap, where the first syllable collapses into the gap with its own particular characteristics. The diver entering the water and reaching the bottom of his dive corresponds to the second stage, where the first syllable is destroyed and there is a state of non-activity. For a brief moment the diver is between descending and coming up. This corresponds to the third stage of lively possibilities, before the diver has taken a particular angle of ascent. Finally the diver comes out. This is the last stage. Even though it is the same diver, having gone through the dive he comes out feeling different (e.g., he feels fresher, the water has had a cooling effect on his mind and body). Similarly, consciousness moving within

The Four Stages of the Gap within the Self-Interacting Dynamics of Consciousness

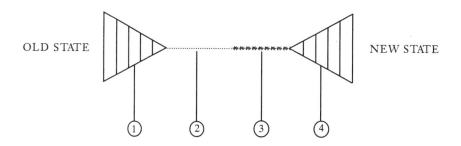

1. PRADHVANSABHAV: **Collapse of old state.**
2. ATYANTABHAV: **Non-activity, unmanifest silence.**
3. ANYONYABHAV: Lively **transformation or self-interaction.**
4. PRAGABHAV: **Emergence of following structure of natural law (new state).**

Maharishi has identified four stages of the gap between two expressions of natural law in the Ved. The first is the collapse of the previous state, pradhvansabhav. The second is a stage of non-activity or unmanifest silence, atyantabhav. Next is a stage of lively transformations or self-interacting dynamics—anyonyabhav. These dynamics structure the fourth stage, pragabhav, the emergence of the following structure of natural law.

itself undergoes a sequential transformation.

The particular quality and dynamics of each gap are determined by the syllables on either side—the initial state that is transformed and the end state that is created. Thus different dynamics of natural law are lively in different gaps between the sounds of the Ved.

This blueprint of the sequential unfoldment of the Ved is referred to by the Sanskrit word *smriti*, which means "memory." The principle of memory upholding the sequential unfoldment of pure knowledge in the Ved is remarkably similar to the faculty of memory in DNA, which ensures that the entire sequential unfoldment of biological information occurs with orderliness and coherence.

The First Sukt of Rik Ved

Now that we understand the overall structure of the Ved, and especially the importance of the gaps, we can appreciate Maharishi's detailed analysis of the beginning sections of Rik Ved, as shown in the Constitution of the Universe chart

Earlier we mentioned the different component parts in which the Rik Ved is organized. The smallest units are syllables. Eight syllables make up a *pad*. Three padas constitute a *richa* (a line or verse), which thus contains 24 syllables. The first nine richas of the Rik Ved form the first *sukt*. The first 192 suktas comprise the first *mandal*—defined in Maharishi's Vedic Science as a "circular cyclical eternal structure." In Rik Ved, there are ten mandalas.

Another important feature of Maharishi's analysis of the gaps in Rik Ved is that the specific mechanics of transformation in each gap is elaborated by specific expressions and sections of the Ved that follow.

Maharishi explains that the first syllable of the Ved, AK, contains the total dynamics of consciousness knowing itself. According to Maharishi's Apaurusheya Bhashya of the Ved, AK describes the collapse of fullness of consciousness (A) within itself to its own point value (K). This collapse, which represents the eternal dynamics of consciousness knowing itself, occurs in eight successive stages. In the next stage of unfoldment of the Ved, these eight stages of collapse are separately elaborated in the eight syllables of the first pad. The first pad thus emerges from, and provides a further commentary on, the first syllable of Rik Ved, AK. These eight syllables correspond to the

The First Section of the Constitution of the Universe Chart, Showing the First Eight Syllables of the First Eight Richas Comprising the First Sukt of Rik Ved

Ahamkar	Buddhi	Manas	Akash	Vayu	Agni	Jal	Prithivi
ऋक्	नि	मी	ळे	पु	रो	हिं	तं
AK	NI	MI	LE	PU	RO	HI	TAM
अ	ग्निः	पू	वैं	भि	ऋ	षि	भि
अ	ग्नि	ना	र	यि	म	श्न	व
अ	गे	यं	यु	ज्ञ	म	ध्व	रं
अ	ग्नि	हों	ता	कृ	वि	कं	तुः
य	द	ज्ञं	दा	शु	षे	तु	वं
उ	प	त्वा	ग्रे	दि	वे	दि	वे
रा	ज	न्त	म	ध्व	रा	षां	गो
स	नः	पि	ते	व	सु	न	वे

eight *prakritis*, or eight fundamental qualities of intelligence, which Maharishi explains constitute "the divided nature of pure conscious-ness." (The eight prakritis—*Ahamkar*, etc.—are listed across the top of the chart. They include the five tanmatras—Akash, Vayu, etc.—discussed in Chapter 5.)

Maharishi's analysis of how the Rik Ved unfolds from this point on brings out further levels of detail. In general, what happens is that all the succeeding padas, richas, and suktas of Rik Ved emerge from the specific mechanics of transformation—the unmanifest, eight-fold structure—in the various gaps between the syllables in the first sukt. Also, the three padas (phrases of eight syllables) in each richa (line) express the eight prakritis with respect to the Rishi, Devata, and Chhandas qualities of pure consciousness. A more detailed and com-plete description of the various stages of elaboration in the Rik Ved is given in the following table.

Stages of Elaboration of Rik Ved

- The **first line, or richa, of the first sukt,** comprising **24 syllables,** provides a further commentary on the **first pad (phrase of 8 syllables)**: the 8-syllable structure of the first pad now appears 3 times.

  - The **first pad** expresses the 8 prakritis (fundamental qualities of intelligence) with respect to the **knower** or **Rishi** quality of pure consciousness.
  - The **second pad** expresses the 8 prakritis with respect to the **process of knowing** or **Devata** (dynamism) quality of pure consciousness.
  - The third pad expresses the 8 prakritis with respect to the **known** or **Chhandas** quality of pure consciousness.
  - Together, these **3 padas** comprise the **first richa (verse)** of the Ved, which represents another complete stage in the sequential unfoldment of knowledge.

- The **subsequent 8 lines** complete the remainder of the first sukt—the next stage of sequential unfoldment of knowledge in the Ved.

  - These 8 lines consist of **24 padas (phrases),** comprising **8 x 24 = 192 syllables.**
  - According to Maharishi's Apaurusheya Bhashya, these **24 padas of 8 syllables** elaborate the unmanifest, 8-fold structure of the **24 gaps between the syllables** of the first richa (verse).

- Each line consists of **3 padas** which, as in the first richa, respectively present the structure of self-interaction with respect to **Rishi** (observer), **Devata** (dynamism quality—process of observation), and **Chhandas** (observed) qualities of pure consciousness.

- Ultimately, in subsequent stages of unfoldment, these **192 syllables of the first sukt (stanza)** get elaborated in the **192 suktas that comprise the first mandal** of the Rik Ved,* which in turn gives rise to the rest of the Ved and the entire Vedic literature.

* The manifest 191 suktas in the first mandala of Rik Ved plus one *avyakt* or "unmanifest" sukt. This unmanifest sukt is one of Maharishi's many significant discoveries, for it completes the total structure of the Ved.

The next figure shows the full significance of the stages of elaboration in Maharishi's Apaurusheya Bhashya, in the context of the whole of Rik Ved, and in the broader context of the entire Samhita of the Ved.

Total Potential of Natural Law in its Most Concentrated Form in the Self

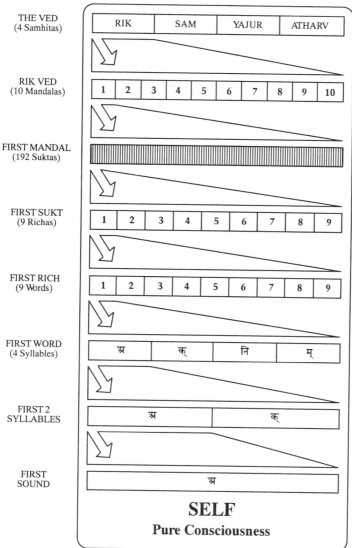

THE VED (4 Samhitas)	RIK	SAM	YAJUR	ATHARV

| **RIK VED** (10 Mandalas) | 1 | 2 | 3 | 4 | 5 | 6 | 7 | 8 | 9 | 10 |

FIRST MANDAL (192 Suktas)

| **FIRST SUKT** (9 Richas) | 1 | 2 | 3 | 4 | 5 | 6 | 7 | 8 | 9 |

| **FIRST RICH** (9 Words) | 1 | 2 | 3 | 4 | 5 | 6 | 7 | 8 | 9 |

| **FIRST WORD** (4 Syllables) | अ | क् | नि | म् |

| **FIRST 2 SYLLABLES** | अ | क् |

| **FIRST SOUND** | अ |

SELF
Pure Consciousness

The total potential of natural law is contained in its concentrated form in the four Samhitas of the Ved, and in increasingly concentrated forms in Rik Ved, in the first mandal of Rik Ved, in the first sukt of the first mandal, in the first richa of the first sukt, in the first word of the first richa, in the first two sounds of the first word, A and K, and in the first sound A. The totality of natural law, contained in each of these expressions, is found in the most concentrated state in the Self, the field of pure consciousness.

The diagram shows how the total potential of natural law is present at every level of the unfoldment of the Ved, from the four Samhitas down to the very first sound of the Rik Ved. And, as the whole of the Ved is found reverberating within pure consciousness, the total potential of natural law is therefore found in its most concentrated form within the Self.

Maharishi explains that the Ved is the internal structure or fabric of consciousness. In Maharishi's words, it "quantifies" the infinite, eternal wholeness of consciousness. The simplest and most fundamental quantification of these dynamics is the three-in-one structure, the Samhita of Rishi, Devata, and Chhandas. All the succeeding transformations are permutations of this basic structure of knowledge, which is reverberating within the Self of everyone.

Rik: Expression of the Total Reality of Dynamic Silence

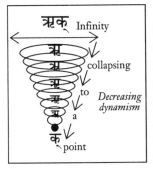

In recent years Maharishi's deep insight into his Apaurusheya Bhashya of Rik Ved has uncovered the dynamics of natural law displayed in its name, which he explains means the "Ved of Rik—knowledge of Rik." Referring to the Sanskrit letters for the sounds comprising the word Rik, he explains that "Rik is a word whose pronunciation displays dynamism from infinity to a point—ऋऋऋऋऋऋऋक् (RRRRRRRR) displays dynamism and क् (K) displays stop of dynamism. क् (K) is a syllable whose pronunciation stops the flow of speech; क् (K) stops the flow of speech."

Maharishi's description of the structure of Rik is shown in the diagrams. He describes the structure of Rik as the dynamics of the relationship between ऋऋऋऋऋऋऋक् (RRRRRRRR) and क् (K), which display "the collapse of dynamism" and the "unfoldment of increasing silence." As he explains, "The relationship between ऋऋऋऋऋऋऋक् (RRRRRRRR) and क् (K) displays the collapse of dynamism to a point. This collapse of dynamism amounts to unfoldment of increasing silence, until the silence becomes infinite at the point."

Thus, Maharishi explains, "The structure of Rik, as displayed in the word Rik, stands for collapse of dynamism to a point and rise of silence

244

from point to infinity, presenting the total reality of all transformations from infinity to a point and point to infinity." And thus the Rik Ved is the Ved of "all possible transformations of the eternal dynamism aspect of the ultimate reality and also of all possible transformations of the eternal silent aspect of the ultimate reality." Rik Ved presents "total reality as the dynamic silence."

Maharishi emphasizes that this level of reality is "the eternally silent potential of all dynamism," and that it is available to everyone in his own transcendental consciousness "where consciousness is fully awake in its pure wakefulness":

> When human awareness settles it identifies itself with this level of reality (Rik Ved). In its pure wakefulness, it not only comprehends the details of interaction between silence and dynamism which form the total mechanics of creation within itself, but at the same time it is the lively potentiality of dynamism in its eternally silent nature.

Maharishi's unique insight into the structure of Rik gives us a vision of the great riches of knowledge and experience in store for us through Maharishi's Vedic Science as we evolve towards higher states of consciousness. This is the knowledge of the laws of nature at the basis of creation, which are eternally lively in their dynamic silence in our own field of pure consciousness—the knowledge that, in Maharishi's words, "is competent to create perfection in all areas of life":

> It is this reality that makes human consciousness the expression of pure knowledge, the Ved—lively field of all possibilities. Maharishi's Vedic Science is the science of this level of reality that is competent to create perfection in all areas of life, because life is an expression of unified wholeness of total reality.

Support of Nature: Practical Benefit of Enlivening the Constitution of the Universe

Now that we have seen the structure of the Rik Ved in more detail, we can understand better why Maharishi has called it the Constitution of the Universe. And fortunately for everyone, Maharishi's Vedic Science and Technology provides not only detailed intellectual understanding of the Constitution of the Universe, but a highly practical, scientifically validated technology to apply this most fundamental and powerful level of natural law for the benefit of mankind.

Maharishi has said that the Constitution of the Universe is lively in "the intelligence of every grain of creation," in every part and in every holistic value of the universe, and in human physiology. By making use of the infinite organizing power of the Constitution of the Universe, he emphasizes, every single individual and every group of individuals and every nation can enjoy full support of natural law.

In our age of modern science, we think of the laws of physics as the most fundamental expression of the laws of nature. In Maharishi's Vedic Science, however, the primordial sounds of the Vedic literature are a far more fundamental expression of these laws. In modern science, the laws can be understood only through intellectual analysis. Through Maharishi's Vedic Science, the laws can be understood both through intellectual analysis and through direct experience. The inner experience of these laws of nature takes place as a result of refining our nervous system so that it can support the experience of higher states of consciousness through Maharishi's Transcendental Meditation and TM-Sidhi program.

On the level of the intellect, Maharishi teaches that the Vedic literature provides us with the knowledge that everything in the universe is an expression of the self-interacting dynamics of pure consciousness. On the level of direct experience, we know that the Constitution of the Universe is fully awake in the field of pure consciousness, which is nothing other than our own simplest state of awareness—our own Self. Without this direct experience, all of Vedic knowledge would be merely another philosophical discourse.

By now, it should be obvious that Maharishi's explanation of the structure and sequence of Rik Ved is light years beyond those given by any other commentators in the East or West. His unique insight has penetrated to the deepest level of meaning of these sounds. As countless translations have demonstrated, the words, phrases, and sections of the Vedic literature do have meaning at the surface level of the intellect. However, because the deeper layers of meaning embedded in the structure of sound and silence in the Ved have been lost to view, these waking-state translations have presented at best a confusing mixture of stories, which through the centuries have become clouded with superstition and understood mainly as myths—a result of their deep significance having been fundamentally misunderstood. Fortunately, the

246

deepest level of their meaning has been available to the supremely enlightened intellect of Maharishi, who has restored the full dignity of the ancient Vedic wisdom; his great gift to humanity has been to make widely available both this understanding, and the technology through which anyone can come to experience the Ved, the primordial sounds of natural law, in one's own consciousness.

In fact, not only *can* we do this, but it is vital and necessary to human life that we do so. For this is the great *practical* benefit to human life of using the technologies of consciousness Maharishi has brought to light from the Vedic literature to gain access to the Constitution of the Universe: support of all the laws of nature. When the Constitution of the Universe is fully lively in our awareness, then life is lived in accord with all the laws of nature governing physiological, psychological, and sociological processes. As a result, problems of ill health and inappropriate behavior do not arise. We receive the support of all the laws of nature for the fulfillment of our desires and aspirations, and for a healthy and happy life.

Brahm, the Charioteer of All Activity

Support of the government of nature is a very real phenomenon. To explain the basis of support of nature, Maharishi often quotes the following verse from Rik Ved describing how *Brahm*—the supreme cosmic intelligence, the infinite organizing power of nature—becomes "the charioteer of all activity"—the prime mover of life:

Yatinam Brahma bhavati sarathih
(Rik Ved 1.158.6)

For those who are established in the singularity of fully awake, self-referral consciousness, Brahm, the Creator—the infinite organizing power of natural law—becomes the charioteer of all activity.

Maharishi explains how success in any activity stems from the principle of "spontaneous administration," which lies in developing "fully awake, self-referral consciousness." This results when the experience of transcendental consciousness is stabilized through regular practice of his Transcendental Meditation and TM-Sidhi program:

Fully awake, self-referral state of consciousness is just the stabilized quality of transcendental consciousness, which is available to anyone

247

through regular practice of my Transcendental Meditation and TM-Sidhi program.

Maharishi explains the mechanics of support of nature: how it is "activity promoted by the infinite organizing power of the unified field," and how this is available to anyone—to individuals and even whole nations—in their own pure consciousness through the technologies of consciousness:

> Activity promoted by pure consciousness is the activity upheld by the infinite organizing power of the unified field (Samhita) of natural law.
>
> This is commonly known as "support of nature," because not knowing the principle of success through one's action, one thinks that one is supported by powers outside oneself, but in fact the phenomenon of support of nature is the phenomenon of one's own pure consciousness—self-referral consciousness
>
> Now is the time when the mechanics of support of nature have been completely understood, and support of nature can not only be gained by the individual, by developing pure consciousness through Transcendental Meditation, but can even be gained by national consciousness, the collective consciousness of the nation, through collective practice (group practice) of the Transcendental Meditation and TM-Sidhi program.
>
> In scientific terminology, support of nature is called life according to natural law, life according to the Constitution of the Universe.

In this context, commenting on *Yatinam Brahma bhavati sarathih*, Maharishi places emphasis on the concept expressed by the word *yatinam*, which refers to "those who are established in self-referral consciousness." Maharishi emphasizes the importance of many people in every nation becoming "yatis"—that is, people who are established in self-referral consciousness. When self-referral consciousness is well established in the collective consciousness of groups of many people (through the Maharishi Effect), then not only for the individual people themselves, but for the whole nation, will Brahm drive the chariot of life.

Training in this field, Maharishi emphasizes, should be "the sole focus of education":

> The enlivenment of the structure of pure knowledge in the Self is and should be the sole focus of education, the sole focus of training whereby the total organizing power inherent in the Self is kept lively

all the time so that the whole force, the whole impetus of organizing anything is coming from that total potential of natural law within one-self. The support of nature for one's thoughts and desires—this ability to have the thoughts and desires come out fully supported by natural law must be enlivened through education.

This supreme level of education is the purpose and goal of the Maharishi Vedic Universities Maharishi has established on every conti-nent. In his recent book, *Maharishi's Absolute Theory of Government*, Maharishi describes how this Vedic Science based education will "infuse the self-referral quality in the collective consciousness of the nation," which will raise the functioning of the government to be "on a par with the government of nature":

> On the practical level it only amounts to introducing my Transcen-dental Meditation and my Vedic Science and Technology, the science and technology of consciousness—the study of consciousness and research in consciousness—in all schools and colleges.
>
> Daily study of consciousness and research in consciousness in the field of education will train the whole population to spontaneously maintain that self-referral quality in individual consciousness, which will infuse the self-referral quality in the collective consciousness of the nation and create the Maharishi Effect.
>
> As national consciousness is the prime mover of the government, when the self-referral quality is lively in national consciousness it will spontaneously render the functioning of the government on a par with the government of nature.

Support of nature, Maharishi explains, is nothing other than living our life in accord with all the laws of nature. Then nature organizes for the fulfillment of our aspirations in a natural and spontaneous way—even sometimes before the desire comes to us. This is like a mother who, recognizing that her child needs a new coat, buys him one before he has even realized that he needs or has formulated the desire for one. Like this, we find that the government of nature spontaneously orga-nizes for the fulfillment of our desires. The environment supports us. On the basis of our fully-awake, blissful self-referral consciousness within, our mind-body behavior conducts itself more fluidly and more gracefully. This is the administration of the government of nature, and the practical benefits of this are unprecedented and very great. As Maharishi said at the time of his discovery of the Constitution of the

Universe, "the scientific knowledge of the source of nature's perfect functioning" has given us the means to develop perfection in life:

> We are now in possession of that supreme knowledge of natural law—the scientific knowledge of the source of nature's perfect order and how to access it—that can bestow perfection on any individual and on any government, and can raise life everywhere to the level of Heaven on Earth.

With the technologies of Maharishi's Vedic Science, we are able to discover the Constitution of the Universe, in Maharishi's phrase, "within the scintillating intelligence of the ever-expanding universe." We are able to repeatedly explore the dynamics of consciousness, of nature's intelligence and creativity that administer our health and physiology, and the entire universe, within our own Self. We are able to maintain the evolution of all the diverse expressions of consciousness in our life—including every aspect of our constantly changing bodies—on the basis of their connectedness with their source in the self-referral, silent state of unity, in the singularity of our own unbounded pure consciousness. We are able to say, not "I *know* the Ved," but "I *am* the Ved." In this way, we are able to bring perfection to our life. This is the ultimate significance of the Ved. As Maharishi explains,

> Ved is the reality of the unified field, where consciousness is in its self-referral state. In that self-referral state of consciousness, different activities come out as a result of the self-interaction of pure consciousness. In this we have the key to all possibilities in human awareness. Human awareness is just the expression of the Self within. Self is a lively field of all the laws of nature. This is the connection of the Ved with the individual and with the universe.

15

DNA AND VED

BRIGHT LIGHTS SHONE ON THE SOFTLY COLORED FLOWERS that surrounded Maharishi. For several hours we had been absorbed in a discussion of how DNA expresses the qualities of the Ved.

"DNA in its innocence," Maharishi explained, "sits there awake to its holistic nature. Then whatever is required, the environment draws from it. Whatever is necessary the environment draws from it. The whole environment is the creation of DNA."

Maharishi explained that this property of DNA was very similar to the Ved, in which the whole infinite range of natural law is fully awake at every point of intelligence, and how this "wakefulness" quality of DNA allows it to respond to the need of the environment: "In the Ved everything is available at each point. The whole range of infinity is fully awake at each point of intelligence. . . . The wakefulness quality of DNA is like the resource of all possibilities, fully awake in itself. It is like that situation which is expressed in words, knock and the door will open. DNA responds to the requirement of the environment, whatever is needed. DNA is a particle of intelligence, a beautiful gift of all possibilities to this human structure."

The discussion continued on. Like many similar meetings before, it resulted in a remarkable integration of knowledge between modern physiology and Vedic physiology. Maharishi's Vedic Physiology, as I explained at the beginning of this book, is the study of physiology in the light of the unified state of pure consciousness. It encompasses all levels: the physiology of consciousness, the physiology of matter, the physiology of society, and the physiology of the universe. Each level is examined with reference to the knowledge and experience of the self-interacting dynamics of consciousness within the unified field at the basis of nature.

What are the textbooks of Maharishi's Vedic Physiology? Because it is a part of Maharishi's Vedic Science, naturally we would expect our study of it to draw heavily on the main sources of knowledge—the Rik Ved and the Vedic literature—we have become familiar with in the last few chapters. But what about modern scientific texts about the body?

Maharishi's Vedic Science includes both the objective approach of modern science and the subjective approach of the ancient Vedic tradition. It is a comprehensive knowledge of life. By studying modern physiology in the light of the knowledge of the Ved, the whole discipline becomes greatly enriched. But the difference between Vedic and modern physiology is also one of emphasis. Vedic Physiology gives first consideration to the fundamental transformations of natural law, the rules that govern all the mechanics of the unified field—in other words, the Constitution of the Universe. It then studies how these transformations are expressed in the manifest universe, how they create the various hierarchical layers of life, including the human physiology.

Scientists have worked closely with Maharishi over many years to develop and explore this field of knowledge from different angles of research. In the course of this continuing research project, many fruitful lines of discussion have emerged examining closely the transition point between consciousness and matter, which we've seen is a major topic in Maharishi's Vedic Science.

These lines of research and discussion have proceeded into the present time, inspired by Maharishi and often catalyzed by his deep insights not only into the Vedic literature but also into the finer areas of modern scientific disciplines. As they have developed, parallels have emerged between modern physiology and Maharishi's Vedic Physiology, which illustrate this close connection between consciousness and matter.

DNA, the Ved of the Body

As the universe is an expression of the knowledge of the Ved, the body is an expression of the knowledge contained in DNA. In Chapter 6 we briefly discussed the connection between DNA and the Ved. DNA stands as the "unified field" of our physiology. Every cell of our body contains DNA molecules, and inscribed within this molecule is the information that specifies every aspect of physiological structure and function. DNA is the medium in which the knowledge of life is recorded. This information is then transcribed and translated by RNA into the numerous protein molecules that help regulate all the bio-chemical and physiological activity in our body.

Maharishi has described how DNA embodies the administration of nature, in that all of the expressions of DNA in the physiology evolve and progress on the basis of being nourished by and remaining connected to their source in the silent, self-referral quality of DNA. Maharishi further explains how perfect governmental administration—a theme he has recently been emphasizing—must be based on the same silent, self-referral functioning of nature that is seen within "the pattern of functioning of DNA":

> The administration in nature is demonstrated in the functioning of DNA, which promotes RNA (various types) in an ever-evolving mood until the impulse of knowledge—the impulse of consciousness (RNA)—transforms itself into material particles (protein) and continues to evolve into the different aspects of the physiology.
>
> In this way every particle of the physiology is always enjoying evolution by virtue of its connectedness with its source, the DNA.
>
> If ever the administration of any government is to be perfect it can only be, it must be, within the pattern of the functioning of DNA. Silent DNA, pulsating within itself, . . . remaining eternally self-referral, spontaneously offers nourishment to all its expressions and inspires all its expressions—every fiber of the physiology—to remain self-referral.
>
> Everything is administered by virtue of its connectedness with its source, which is self-sufficient, invincible, pure intelligence.

Maharishi's Apaurusheya Bhashya of the Ved describes how the knowledge in the Ved unfolds in an orderly, systematic pattern. The Ved begins with an expression of wholeness of knowledge, and each succeeding verse provides a commentary on the preceding ones. When the sequential elaboration of knowledge is complete, there is a return to the wholeness of the original expression. Maharishi explains that the content of each of the four Vedas takes the form of a cyclical pattern which embodies this sequential elaboration of knowledge and return to wholeness. These cyclical patterns take the form of *mandalas* which I referred to in the previous chapter as major divisions of knowledge in the Vedas. Mandalas, Maharishi explains, are a series of circle-like structures, which naturally order and preserve the information contained in them.

Each DNA molecule also has a form that naturally orders and preserves information. The physical structure of DNA consists of the well-known "double helix"—an arrangement of carbon, hydrogen, oxygen, nitrogen, and phosphorus atoms woven together in two complementary strands. The complementary double helical structure of DNA was discovered in 1953 by James B. Watson and Francis Crick, who subsequently won the Nobel prize for their discovery.

Information is coded within DNA through the sequence of specific chemicals called nucleotides. A strand of DNA contains a specific sequence of four nucleotide bases: adenosine (A), thymosine (T), guanosine (G), and cytosine (C). The four nucleotide bases are the fundamental letters of the genetic alphabet (A, T, G, C). They may be compared to the fundamental sounds or syllables that are the elementary components of the Ved. The letters along the DNA strand form words that consist of three nucleotides, such as ATC. Since there are only four letters in the DNA alphabet, the total number of possible combinations of three-letter words is actually 64. This is technically a larger number than is needed to code for the 20 amino acids that are the building blocks of all proteins. However, some of the words are duplicates for the same amino acid; others serve as "punctuation marks" denoting the beginning or end of a piece of information within the DNA. What is particularly interesting is that if we consider the number of possible combinations, 64, from the Vedic Physiology perspective of Rishi, Devata, and Chhandas, we then have three permutations of the 64 possible words, making 192 possible combinations in all.

This corresponds to the 192 syllables in the first sukt of Rik Ved and to the 192 suktas of the first mandal.

This observation was first made by three noted scientists and physicians, Dr. Roger Chalmers, Dr. Tony Nader, and Dr. Hari Sharma, working with Maharishi. It reveals the intimate connection between the Constitution of the Universe and the DNA molecule. Using the language of DNA, the genetic code, it should be possible to follow the example of Dr. Hagelin in physics and outline the detailed correspondence between DNA and the Rik Ved.

The Three-in-One Structure of DNA

What in DNA might correspond to Rishi, Devata, and Chhandas? The unfoldment of information from DNA requires the existence of a completely unified and holistic level of knowledge that silently integrates and coordinates the entire physiology. This is the level of Samhita. In DNA the Samhita level may be thought of as the totality of knowledge containing the complete record or memory of life that is present within the DNA of all living systems.

The Rishi or "knower" value corresponds to the information within DNA that is involved in knowing itself. We may equate this with the intelligence value of DNA, in the silent knowledge that is contained in the physical structure of the molecule.

The Devata or "process of knowing" value corresponds to the organizing power inherent within DNA, which has the ability to initiate and govern biological transformations. Contained in seed form within DNA is the entire range of possible transformations that give rise to the enormous diversity of life.

The Chhandas or "known" value corresponds to the information within DNA that delineates its physical structure. The orderly physical nature of DNA, particularly the precise sequence of nucleotides, is vital for the formation and preservation of the structure of the entire organism.

The values of Rishi, Devata, and Chhandas described in Maharishi's Vedic Science can be seen at all the various levels within the physiology. On the next page is a chart depicting the hierarchical

MAHARISHI'S VEDIC SCIENCE AND TECHNOLOGY
UNIFIED FIELD CHART FOR PHYSIOLOGY

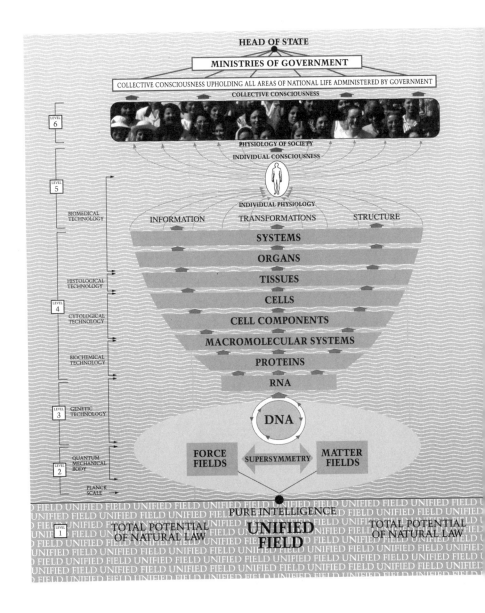

organization of the human physiology. The three streams of Rishi, Devata, and Chhandas can be located in terms of information, transformations, and structure at all levels from DNA to cells and finally to the various systems of the body.

A detailed parallel between the Vedic literature and physiology can be seen in a model developed by Dr. John Fagan, professor of molecular biology and co-director of the doctoral program in physiology at Maharishi International University. Working with Maharishi, he has correlated the three-in-one structure of DNA with specific branches of Vedic literature. For example, he has drawn a parallel between the genome, the totality of genetic information contained in an organism, and the Brahmanas. As we have seen, the Brahmanas are described by Maharishi as displaying the infinite organizing power of the Ved. Likewise, the genome can be understood as the organizing power for a particular organism. It specifies every aspect of biochemical, cellular, and organismic structure and function.

In this model, the organizing power of the Brahmanas is compared with the organizing power of the genome of a specific organism. This model is further elaborated by examining the three-in-one structure of the Brahmanas and the genome. We recall that *Brahmanas* refers both collectively to three aspects of the Vedic literature—the Upanishads, the Aranyakas, and the Brahmanas—as well as to the last of these three by itself.

Maharishi has explained that in the sequential unfoldment of the Ved, the Upanishads present the details of the nature of the Rishi, the underlying notion of the subject, the Self. The Aranyakas focus on the Devata value, the process of knowing. The Brahmanas elaborate on the Chhandas value, the object of knowing. The Brahmanas do not exclude the value of the subject or the process of knowing. Rather, they tend to emphasize the practical application of this knowledge in the form of specific procedures, *yagyas*, which we described in Chapter 6. Yagyas are designed to enliven specific mechanics of transformation at the level of pure consciousness to produce specific life-supporting effects on the manifest level of life, as a means to bring life in accordance with natural law. The Rishi, Devata, and Chhandas aspects of the genome are described in terms of these three branches of the Vedic literature.

Correspondence of the Upanishads, Aranyakas, and Brahmanas with Rishi, Devata and Chhandas and with Different Aspects of DNA

In Dr. Fagan's model (see figure on next page), the Upanishads (Rishi) correspond to the information specifying the mechanisms by which a particular organism preserves and perpetuates the biological information carried in its genome. Level One in the figure shows that this class includes all information that directs the processes of DNA replication and DNA repair. DNA replication duplicates the genome in preparation for cell division; DNA repair restores information at risk due to chemical alteration of the DNA. The information governing these processes can be further subdivided (Level Two in the figure). For example, the process of replication includes: (a) Rishi—replication signals (such as the class of signals known as "origins of replication"); (b) Devata—the genes, or blueprints, for enzymes that mediate the process of replication (e.g., DNA polymerase); and (c) Chhandas—the replicated genome itself.

The Aranyakas (Devata) correspond to all information specifying the mechanics through which the information contained within the genome can be altered. This class of biological information (Level One) includes that which directs the processes of genomic rearrangement, recombination, and mutation. Each of these processes involves the reorganization of information in DNA. The information governing each of these processes can be further subdivided (Level Two). For instance, in the process of recombination we find the following: (a) Rishi—"recombination signals," those DNA sequences within the genome that provide the information to direct the recombination of DNA; (b) Devata—the genes that encode the enzymes, the biological catalysts that mediate recombination; and (c) Chhandas—the new organization of genetic information in the genome, which is the result or outcome of the recombination process.

The Brahmanas (Chhandas) correspond to (Level One) all information specifying biological structures and functions and all information governing their process of expression. The three subclasses of biological information (Level Two) that can be identified at this level are: (a) Rishi—DNA sequences that function as control signals for any

The Self-Interacting Dynamics of Rishi, Devata, and Chhandas at the Level of the Brahmanas in the Vedic Literature and the Genome in Molecular Biology

Vedic Literature	Self-Interacting Dynamics of Consciousness	Molecular Biology
Brahmanas		**Genome**

Upanishads

Rishi knower

Level One—All information specifying: mechanisms by which the organism *preserves and perpetuates* biological information in its genome (e.g., DNA replication and repair).

Level Two: DNA replication
- *Rishi* — replication signals
- *Devata* — genes for enzymes that mediate replication
- *Chhandas* — replicated genome

Aranyakas

Devata process of knowing

Level One—All information specifying: mechanics through which information in the genome can be *altered* (e.g., rearrangement, recombination, and mutation).

Level Two: Recombination
- *Rishi* — recombination signals
- *Devata* — genes for enzymes mediating recombination
- *Chhandas* — new organization of information in genome

Brahmanas

Chhandas known

Level One—All information specifying: *biological structures and functions* and their *processes of expression.*

Level Two: Gene expression
- *Rishi* — DNA sequences that function as control signals
- *Devata* — genes encoding enzymes that catalyze steps of expression
- *Chhandas* — sequences specifying biological structures

259

aspect of the process of gene expression (including transcriptional control sequences such as promoters, operators, and enhancers, and mRNA processing signals); (b) Devata—the genes encoding the enzymes that catalyze the steps of gene expression (including the genes for RNA polymerase and for splicing and capping enzymes, and those encoding repressors and apoinducers, which are specific proteins that regulate gene expression); and (c) Chhandas—the sequences specifying the actual structures of the components of biological systems (including enzymes, structural proteins, peptide hormones, ribosomal RNAs, and transfer RNAs).

Smriti and DNA:
The Precise, Sequential Unfoldment of Knowledge

As we saw in Chapter 13, in the self-interacting dynamics of pure consciousness which constitute the Ved and the Vedic literature, the totality of pure knowledge responsible for the entire manifest creation is contained in the form of *smriti*, or "memory." Maharishi explains that the smriti value of the Ved ensures the precise sequential unfoldment of knowledge from the unified field.

We can also find a smriti value in DNA. The knowledge represented in the DNA molecules of every cell in every living creature may be considered the record, or "memory," of millions of years of biological adaptation and evolution. This memory also contains the information necessary for further adaptation and evolution of new organisms.

The complete plan for the human body, as we have seen, exists within the memory of DNA. Like an architect's blueprint or a computer program, the genetic information contained in DNA encodes the instructions for building and maintaining each system. The human brain, for example, has over one hundred billion cells, all interconnected in the most complex patterns. How does each cell know how to contact another?

In the process of development, specific regions of information in the memory of DNA begin to be sequentially expressed. When a young, unspecialized cell develops into a mature cell (such as a neuron or white blood cell capable of performing a particular function), there is a sequential expression of information from the totality of biological intelligence in the DNA of the cell.

This process is known as cell differentiation. Each cell comes to perform a specialized function, while yet maintaining the memory of the knowledge organizing the life history of the entire organism. Each differentiated cell contributes to the welfare of the whole organism, while it also benefits from the increased complexity of the whole organism.

The timing of the expression of genetic information governs the sequential development of an undifferentiated cell to a fully differentiated, mature cell. Evidence indicates that specific regulatory regions on the DNA are turned on and off in a particular sequence during the process of development. Several regulatory proteins may be produced from DNA which in turn interact with it, inducing the synthesis of a new set of regulatory proteins characteristic of the next stage of development. The synthesis of these regulatory proteins is induced by the interaction of a previous set of regulatory proteins with DNA. Ultimately an initial protein or primordial set of proteins may be located which begins the entire process of cellular development.

The initial, primordial set of proteins in the biological organism is similar to 'A'—the first sound of Rik Ved, the most comprehensive expression of the totality of natural law, from which the rest of the Ved unfolds. We can see in this whole phenomenon a process similar to the self-interacting dynamics of consciousness—the permutations and combinations of Rishi, Devata, and Chhandas referring back to the Samhita, as the Ved sequentially unfolds from within pure consciousness. This again reminds us of the verse from the Bhagavad-Gita: *Prakritim svam avashtabhya visrijami punah punah*, "taking recourse to my own self-referral nature, I create again and again."

It will be illuminating to uncover the principles and dynamics of the expression of biological information during the development of an entire organism in the light of Maharishi's Vedic Physiology, and in particular Maharishi's description of the sequential elaboration of knowledge from its first expressions. For example, the principle that knowledge hidden in the gaps between syllables and richas of the Ved is manifested in subsequent expressions of the Ved may alert researchers to look for sequences of nucleotides, or intervals between sequences, which are "silent" (inactive) at certain stages of development, but convey information at later stages.

A concerted effort is being made by a number of laboratories today to sequence the entire human genome. Before long, ten percent of the genome may be known. From what has emerged so far, it appears that only a small percentage of the nucleotides of the human genome vary from individual to individual. With full knowledge of the human genome from modern science and complete comprehension of the dynamics of the expression of natural law from Maharishi's Vedic Physiology, it should be possible to fully understand the fundamental principles and processes associated with the proper expression of genetic information and the mechanics of how to permanently enliven the memory of a perfectly functioning physiology.

The Richo Akshare Verse of Rik Ved:
The First Principle of Nature's Functioning

Maharishi explains that the "master key" to unfolding the totality of Vedic literature is contained in a single verse of the Rik Ved:

> *Richo akshare parame vyoman*
> *yasmin deva adhivishve nisheduh*
> *yastanna ved kimricha karishyati*
> *ya ittadvidus ta ime samasate*
> Rik Ved (I.164.39)

The verses of the Ved exist in the collapse of fullness (the *kshar* of 'A') in the transcendental field, self-referral consciousness, the Self.

In which reside all the devas, the impulses of creative intelligence, the laws of nature responsible for the whole manifest universe.

He whose awareness is not open to this field, what can the verses accomplish for him?

Those who know this level of reality are established in evenness, wholeness of life.

In Maharishi's explanation, this verse locates the fundamental dynamics of nature's creativity and the source of all expressions of natural law in pure consciousness, the unified field, and explains how the knowledge and experience of pure consciousness bring life to fulfillment.

The first half of this verse presents the theme of self-referral and sequential transformation by which pure consciousness unfolds itself into infinite diversity. The second half of the verse presents the supreme value to human life of the direct experience of these mechanics.

Maharishi has pointed out that the dynamics of natural law expressed in this key verse are expressed in the fundamental theories of every discipline, profession, and trade. We will interpret these dynamics of natural law in the Richo Akshare verse from the viewpoint of modern physiology, thus illuminating the development and application of physiology with reference to its source in the field of pure consciousness.

Richo akshare: First principle of nature's functioning

The first word of the verse, *richo*, means the verses (richas) of the Ved. As we have discussed, the verses are not to be understood in terms of the superficial meaning of their words. We know them from Maharishi's explanation as the fundamental reverberations of consciousness—the deepest level of the laws of nature. The second word, *akshare*, describes how these fundamental expressions of natural law emerge. They emerge from the *kshar of 'A'*, that is, from the collapse of fullness to its point value. The kshar of A, or collapse of A, as we have discussed in the previous chapter, describes the inherent dynamics of the field of pure consciousness, from which emerge the Ved and everything in creation. The expression *richo akshare* identifies this phenomenon as the first principle of nature's functioning, the source of nature's creativity.

The fundamental mechanics of creativity by which DNA expresses its knowledge also involve a self-interacting process. The expression of biological information, as we have seen earlier, occurs when the totality of information contained in the DNA responds to a specific impulse from its environment. For example, when the level of a particular metabolite is changed in the environment of a cell, the DNA responds: it expresses the specific biological information necessary to produce the appropriate protein that can ensure that the metabolite can be metabolized by the cell.

This process of expression of biological information parallels the mechanics of expression of the verses of the Ved. The expression of biological information corresponds to the verse of the Ved (richa), and the totality of information contained in the DNA corresponds to the fullness of A. In DNA the self-referral process of collapse calls to mind

Maharishi's description at the beginning of the chapter of how, in the Ved, "the whole range of infinity is fully awake at each point of intelligence," and that "the wakefulness quality of DNA is like the resource of all possibilities, fully awake in itself. . . . like that situation . . . , 'knock and the door will open.' DNA responds to the requirement of the environment, whatever is needed." The process involves the ability of the DNA to interact with stimuli from the environment—the environment of the cell which the DNA has, in fact, helped create. In responding to the need of the environment, the total potential of knowledge—all the possibilities for expression in DNA—"collapses" to express the particular point value (the specific mode of its own biological intelligence) required at that moment.

Parame vyoman: The transcendental field of life

The second expression of the Richo Akshare verse, *parame vyoman*, "in the transcendental field, self-referral consciousness, the Self," emphasizes that the kshar of A, the dynamics at the source of all the laws of nature, is located in the transcendental field of pure consciousness.

DNA acts as the transcendental field of the physiology. Although it is dynamic from the perspective of biochemistry, from the perspective of physiological functioning DNA is unchanging, serving as the silent blueprint for the entire physiology. The dynamics of the expression of biological information exist and originate within the transcendental field of DNA.

Yasmin deva adhivishve nisheduh: The intelligence of the universe

Maharishi explains that the connection between the transcendental field of consciousness and the structure of natural law is further elaborated in the next expression of the verse: *yasmin deva adhivishve nisheduh*, "in which reside all the devas, the impulses of creative intelligence, the laws of nature responsible for the whole manifest universe."

The devas are the dynamic, creative aspect of the richas. The devas are the seat of the infinite organizing power of natural law inherent in the richas, the fundamental reverberations of consciousness. As we have seen, this organizing power of natural law not only governs all the diverse phenomena of nature, but actually creates the universe: the physical universe is just the most precipitated expression of the Ved, the self-interacting dynamics of the transcendental field of pure consciousness.

264

Within the structure of the DNA molecule are encoded specific subunits of information called genes. Genes are parallel to the devas: they play the same role as the devas in that they contain within them the ability to direct the formation of many proteins, such as enzymes. The proteins encoded by the genes both direct the basic biochemical pathways that underlie all processes in the body and form fundamental structural units in various cells and tissues. Thus the genes embody the intelligence and organizing power of DNA.

Yastanna ved kimricha karishyati: Plight of the ignorant

The second half of the Richo Akshare verse begins with the expression, *yastanna ved kimricha karishyati,* "He whose awareness is not open to this field, what can the verses accomplish for him?" These words emphasize that the richas have practical value; however, it is not available if our awareness is not open to the transcendental field—that is, if we do not directly experience pure consciousness.

In the physiology, a similar situation occurs when the flow of biological information from DNA is disrupted. For example, when a cell becomes cancerous it is no longer able to express properly the information it holds. As we discussed in Chapter 6, it has lost its memory of how to function in a manner that supports the entire organism. Its only concern is to multiply at an ever-faster rate and spread throughout the organism, eventually causing death.

Ya ittadvidus ta ime samasate: Formula for fulfillment

The concluding expression of the verse, *ya ittadvidus ta ime samasate,* "those who know this level of reality are established in evenness, wholeness of life," describes the immense practical benefits that can be gained through the experience of pure consciousness.

In terms of DNA the optimal state of physiological functioning is one in which there is a fully integrated and unimpeded flow of information from the DNA to all parts of the body. Every component of the physiology is harmoniously integrated with the whole through ideally functioning homeostatic feedback systems.

When there is a coherent expression of information from DNA, then stability and wholeness pervade the physiology through all stages of development. As a result the individual's immune system is strong enough to resist disease and prevent disorder from arising, forming the basis for perfect health and longevity.

The many parallels and correspondences between the structure of DNA and the structure of consciousness should come as no surprise, because ultimately DNA is itself the material expression of the self-interacting dynamics of consciousness. Ultimately, therefore, the most ideal unfoldment of the knowledge in DNA in human life will come through regular practice of Maharishi's Transcendental Meditation and TM-Sidhi program. By enlivening the self-interacting dynamics of nature's functioning from the level of pure consciousness, we enliven in all the expressions of Rishi, Devata, and Chhandas throughout the physiology the memory of their connection to their self-referral source in pure consciousness. We begin to educate the DNA such that the full memory of our genetic potential is uncovered. In the Vedic tradition this is called *smriti labda*, memory regained. Through this self-referral process, the functioning of our DNA administers and supports the experience of enlightenment.

CHAPTER 16

THE VEDIC SCIENTIST

MAHARISHI IS FOND OF TAKING BOAT RIDES, WHETHER ON Lake Lucerne in Switzerland or Lake Tahoe in California. Maharishi's lectures during these excursions have brought out some of the most profound and deep knowledge I have ever experienced. I remember one time when I gained perhaps my clearest understanding of Maharishi's description of the language of the Ved. This was during a boat ride with Maharishi in the spring of 1982, on the Rhine river near Boppard, Germany. On this occasion the physicist Dr. John Hagelin was present and the subject of discussion was the language of nature.

Maharishi explained that if we want to comprehend the Ved, then we must experience it in the language of the Ved itself. As he said, "the Ved must sing its own story; in its original script the Ved is just the whisper of the unified field to itself." Dr. Hagelin pointed out that a similar situation applies in physics: if we try to understand the quantum world from a classical perspective we fail to appreciate its full value; we can gain only an approximation of that reality. In the classical realm we assume that matter and events are concrete, localized, and predictable. In the quantum realm matter is neither solid nor static. It is only a condensation, or a concentrated manifestation of an underlying unmanifest quantum field. In order to understand the quantum world we must use the language of the quantum world. Only then, Dr. Hagelin explained, can we comprehend its complete subtlety and wholeness.

In a similar manner, Maharishi continued, if we want to properly understand and describe the Ved, we can do so only from the level of the experience of higher states of consciousness. We need to experience consciousness interacting with itself. This, Maharishi said, is the most profound language of nature—the Ved—which we come to know when we experience nature at its source.

Once we have the experience of higher states of consciousness, Maharishi continued, it is easier to understand waking state consciousness for what it truly is: a special, limited case of consciousness. Trying to understand intellectually the perspective of higher states of consciousness from the perspective of waking consciousness, without the experience of pure consciousness, may prove discouraging and create a sense of boundaries in the awareness rather growing freedom and fulfillment.

The discussion continued for several more hours. At the end, Maharishi summarized by explaining that each viewpoint is valid on its own level, yet the more comprehensive viewpoints give a fuller picture of nature. He referred to a key concept in the Vedic paradigm, "knowledge is structured in consciousness." On one level, the meaning of this principle is that expressed in the Richo Akshare verse of Rik Ved: that the Ved—pure knowledge—exists in the transcendental field, pure consciousness, the Self. A corollary of that point is that our level of consciousness determines how deeply we can comprehend the Ved, and thus how much knowledge we can gain about the world. So far, our experience of the Ved, and thus our knowledge of the universe, has been limited because we have not had access to higher states of consciousness.

The Role of Experience

For over three hundred years, science has been in a quandary over the "problem" of mind and body. Why? Because it is a dilemma of waking state consciousness. In waking state consciousness we are confined to one viewpoint, which finds expression in one limited language of nature. It is indeed a very limited perspective whose language allows only the experience and understanding of separation between mind and body. The dilemma of waking state consciousness is the dilemma of modern science. In waking consciousness we cannot conceive of a state of pure subjectivity that underlies and creates all objective states of matter, including the body, except in the most superficial intellectual terms.

Only by transcending waking state consciousness, experiencing pure consciousness, and learning the new language of higher states of consciousness can we resolve this dilemma. As we know, pure consciousness is the unified state of knower, process of knowing, and known. From the perspective of this higher state of consciousness, mind and body are completely unified: there can be no separation between them, because the body is simply the objective, concrete expression of the same field of pure subjectivity that gives rise to the mind. The body is the physical form, the further expression of the self-interacting dynamics that creates the mind. Only by applying the technology of natural law, Maharishi's technology of consciousness, can we experience higher states of consciousness and use the full potential of our nervous system.

We know from neurophysiological research that different experiences can influence the structure and functioning of the brain. For example, when two groups of animals are raised in either a "rich" environment (containing many types of stimuli) or a "poor" environment (a standard small wire cage) the effects on the brain are significantly different. The animals living in the rich environment develop bigger and heavier brains (a thicker cerebral cortex) and exhibit increased amounts of a key biochemical communicator, acetylcholine. The most interesting difference, however, is a marked increase in interconnections between nerve cells in the animals living in an enriched environment.

The brain is never static or fixed. It is continually changing. With every experience neurotransmitter levels are increasing or decreasing, receptors are being replaced and neural connections are selectively strengthened or weakened. The structure and function of the brain is just a reflection of who we are. If we allow ourselves to become static and frozen in our personal development, locked into the waking state, then our once dynamic brain looses its dynamism and flexibility. If, on the other hand, we continually refine our neurophysiological functioning through the development of higher states of consciousness, then we will continue to unfold its latent potentialities.

As Maharishi has pointed out, it is a situation of "knock and the door will open"—DNA responds to the needs and the experiences presented by the environment. As we systematically and regularly experience transcendental consciousness, the brain becomes more coherent, more balanced. The results are clear from the myriad improvements seen in those who practice Maharishi's Transcendental Meditation and TM-Sidhi program.

Vedic Perception

The Vedic literature is the record of the experiences of the ancient seers who thousands of years ago developed higher states of consciousness. The records of their experiences are in one sense similar to the records of experiments in modern scientific journals. They are repeatable results based on a systematic and repeatable experiential methodology, an inner technology of consciousness. Their object of inquiry was the laws of nature. Unlike modern scientific experiments, their methodology was subjective, their laboratory pure consciousness.

To have these experiences reliably and systematically, the first Vedic scientists, like any scientists, had to be experts in the appropriate technology, in this case the technology of consciousness. They had to refine the functioning of their nervous systems in order to be able to experience and develop higher states of consciousness. Maharishi explains that the Vedic seers perceived these laws of nature as reverberations of sound—the mantras of the Ved—within their own consciousness. They passed down the knowledge they gained orally from one generation to the next, with the understanding that the actual meaning could be fathomed only if one first achieved higher states of consciousness. However, as we saw in discussing the Richo Akshare verse of Rik Ved, precisely because the Vedic method of gaining knowledge depends on a fully developed nervous system, its main field of knowledge—the experience of the self-interacting dynamics of the Ved—long ago became inaccessible when the procedures to gain higher states of consciousness were not available.

The Vedic literature makes clear that this knowledge was available in its completeness in the ancient Vedic civilization, which, as Maharishi tells us, was a time of Heaven on Earth. At that time many people regularly practiced these technologies and achieved higher states of consciousness: the knowledge of the Ved was the vibrant reality of their daily life. However, Maharishi explains that after many generations living in the goal, the path to the goal—the technology of consciousness—was forgotten. Over the long course of history, as pure consciousness faded from the daily life of the people, the knowledge of the Ved became greatly misunderstood and misinterpreted. The situation was further complicated after the Vedic texts had been written down and eventually translated into other languages. Without the experience of the self-interacting dynamics of consciousness, what remained were only the superficial outer trappings of knowledge. As Maharishi has commented, "the study of the Ved is not through the books of the Ved. . . . The study of the Ved is from what is inscribed in the pure consciousness of the individual student himself." Without the experience of pure consciousness, the student of the Ved could eat only the outer peel of the fruit of knowledge; the sweet fruit inside was unsuspected and therefore left untasted. In this situation, the fullness of life became cramped and daily life become full of suffering.

With Maharishi's restoration of the complete knowledge and experience of the Ved, these technologies have once again become widely available. Now it is possible for anyone to systematically and naturally experience pure consciousness as the ultimate basis of all subjective and objective states, and on that basis to become a Vedic scientist. With the experience of consciousness in its purest and most settled state, we become increasingly familiar with the fine fabrics of our own awareness—with the language of the unified field of natural law. We gain the ability to become Vedic physiologists—to examine directly the physiology of consciousness and to witness the physiology of the universe emerging from the vast sea of consciousness.

Maharishi beautifully describes the capability of a Vedic physiologist: "The Vedic physiologist can cognize the laws of nature directly within his own consciousness. They exist in their most concentrated form within the dynamics of consciousness. It is only necessary to be fully awake in the state of pure consciousness." Maharishi further explains the ensuing process of gaining knowledge of the laws of nature, based on one's having become fully awake in the state of pure consciousness:

> In the fully awake state of pure consciousness, the self-interacting dynamics of consciousness begin to reverberate within one's con-

271

sciousness. The nature of the underlying threads of the fabric of consciousness begin to reveal themselves to themselves. The whole process is beautifully expressed in the Rik Ved, *Yojagara tam richa kamayante*—"He who is awake, the richas, the verses of the Ved, the impulses of natural law seek him out." This is the prerequisite for gaining knowledge of the Ved.

The Vedic physiologist is thus able to directly perceive the innermost threads of consciousness as well as all the more manifest levels of the physiology of consciousness and the physiology of matter.

What would this experience be like? Maharishi several years ago gave a hint of what this Vedic perception would entail. He explained that in this highly developed state of enlightenment, the activity of each of the cells in our body should be apparent to us on the most refined level of hearing, as different voices in our consciousness. We would experience these impulses through the same consciousness—our Self—which is continually transforming itself into those impulses of sound and matter.

In this process, the body would become a kind of cinema cognized in terms of sound and vision as lively unity or Samhita. If any impurity or abnormality happened to exist in our nervous system, then the impulses of consciousness (the sounds) would be out of harmony, or balance, with their "meaning" (that is, their precipitated form as matter). Then the highly discriminative ability of this most subtle perception would be lost.

In this case, the perception would be blurred. We might still hear the "hum" of the impulses of consciousness that structure the eyes, the tongue, the aggregate of cells—but we might not perceive the distinct value of the activity of each cell. But if our physiology were completely free of stress, pure and in balance, then the different values of all expressions of the Ved—the syllables, richas, suktas, etc.—would be distinctly perceived as the mechanics structuring the different values of physiology. As the refined perception characteristic of the highest states of consciousness developed, no aspect of natural law would be out of our comprehension. We would hear the whole sukt and all of its parts, each syllable and at the same time the gaps between the syllables—the very mechanics of transformation within consciousness.

The true Vedic physiologists, from Maharishi's point of view, thus have access to the laws of nature within their own consciousness. They are able to cognize the Ved in terms of their own internal functioning. All this is possible because of the intimate relationship of the Ved with human physiology: one is merely a reflection of the other. The whole of the Ved is found embodied in the whole of human physiology.

Vedic scientists awaken within themselves the realization that located in the simplest form of awareness, their own Self, is the source of nature's creativity, the self-referral dynamics of pure consciousness. As we become Vedic Scientists we experience the self-interacting dynamics of consciousness within ourselves, we come to know consciousness as the prime mover of life. We realize that Vedic Science is the science of our own consciousness: moving within itself, the wholeness of our consciousness creates the apparent diversity of the universe. Our own physiology is the physiology of the universe. Maharishi has described this ultimate realization of Vedic wisdom as embodied in the understanding that the total universe is contained in my Self: the Ved is all that there is, the Self is all that there is. This realization is expressed in the Vedic aphorism, *Aham Brahmasmi*, "I am the unbounded totality; I am everything."

Maharishi

In the Vedic tradition there have always been great individuals who have reached the very highest levels of perfection. Their knowledge and inspiration have always upheld the deep value of the Vedic wisdom. Their lives have determined the direction for generations to come.

Today we are experiencing just such an event in human history. A new knowledge is emerging in this scientific age. The man, scientist and saint, who has brought it forth, is Maharishi.

How was Maharishi able to bring to light the correct practice of this ancient technology of consciousness, which for centuries had been misunderstood? He has always given all credit for this revival of Vedic knowledge to his own teacher, Swami Brahmananda Saraswati, known as Guru Dev, who was one of India's greatest teachers in the Vedic tradition. Late in his life Guru Dev accepted the position of the Shankaracharya of Jyotir Math in the Himalayas, a seat of leadership in the Vedic tradition that traces its descent from Shankara, who was responsible for an earlier complete revival of Vedic wisdom many centuries ago.

"The truth of Vedic wisdom is by its very nature independent of time and can therefore never be lost," Maharishi has written. Yet he describes how the original technology for developing higher states of consciousness was forgotten, not once, but many times throughout history, owing, he says, "to the long lapse of time." This, Maharishi explains, is "the tragedy of knowledge, the tragic fate that knowledge must meet at the hands of ignorance. It is inevitable, because the teaching comes from one level of consciousness and is received at quite a different level. The knowledge of unity must in time shatter on the hard rocks of ignorance."

The nervous system of an enlightened person must be keenly sensitive and extremely refined so that it can naturally and spontaneously experience the dynamics of the unified field of nature's intelligence. Since the time of the ancient Vedic rishis, there have been those who have experienced the unified field in its fullness, and gained enlightenment. At the times when the knowledge of the Ved had been temporarily lost to view, these were the great sages who again brought it to light from the Vedic literature in its full brilliance, to set the course of life to run in the most evolutionary direction to fulfill the high purpose of human existence.

Maharishi absorbed the complete experience and understanding of Vedic wisdom under his teacher's guidance and later began a formal, systematic restoration of it. Through the more than 35 years since, as each new area of Vedic knowledge has been unfolded through Maharishi's research and penetrating vision into the Vedic literature, he has inspired its integration with the latest advances in modern science and its formulation into practical educational programs that can be easily implemented everywhere.

By making available this knowledge and technology, Maharishi has given us the greatest resource on earth, the resource of the inner dynamics of consciousness. We must never lose the "memory" of our inner physiology of consciousness; we must never let our connection with it become weak. It is the source of all our creativity, all our success. It is the source of all the riches of nature.

There is a wonderful story Maharishi tells. A saint crossing a river sees a scorpion in the water and bends down to pick it up and save it. The scorpion stings him and then falls back into the water. The saint tries to save it again, with the same result. After this happens several

274

times the people nearby ask the saint, "Why are you trying to save that scorpion which is stinging you?" He answers, "Just as the nature of the scorpion is to sting, it is my nature to save."

Over the years Maharishi has never stopped giving to the world his precious knowledge of his Vedic Science. Sometimes people have criticized this knowledge, but that has not stopped Maharishi who knows its true value. It is a knowledge that can and is transforming the world from problems and suffering to Heaven on Earth.

Maharishi's genius has extended to many areas of life, but his contribution to physiology and health is particularly significant, since physiology is that one area of life that bridges the divergent realms of subjectivity and objectivity, mind and body, consciousness and matter. The knowledge of Maharishi's Vedic Physiology is emerging in this scientific age as a practical technology of natural law to establish perfect health in the individual and society. What Maharishi did when he brought out from the Vedic literature and began teaching this extraordinary ancient science of physiology in the West was nothing less than the single most important scientific discovery of our age. It heralds the exploration of the greatest frontier of modern science, the understanding and practical application of the dynamics of consciousness.

It is appropriate for the final words of this book to come from Maharishi:

> The Ved has been declaring throughout time: "Amritasya Putrah—O Sons of Immortality." From the field of pure knowledge, the mortal has always been welcomed as the descendant of the Immortal. Modern science in its infancy, playing with the fine particles of nature, discovered the destructive potential of natural law, and has delivered total annihilation at the doorstep of human existence. Now it is high time for modern science in its present state of maturity to repay the debt it owes to life. Vedic Science offers the guiding principle. Vedic knowledge is emerging as the most profound science of life, and offers fulfillment to the human quest for perfection. This is the time for modern science to rise to fulfillment.

Notes and References

General Note for All Chapters Regarding
Pronunciation of Maharishi's Vedic Science Terminology

In the context of discussing Maharishi's Vedic Science and Technology, throughout this book a number of Sanskrit terms are used. Please note that we have decided to adopt the convention of excluding any final, short "a" from transliterations of Sanskrit terms (as in Ved rather than Veda), except in plurals and possessives (e.g., Vedas, doshas). For ease in pronunciation, after a "y," a smaller "a" is used (e.g., vaidya, yagya) to indicate that a short "a" may be pronounced, but with less emphasis. This is the convention used by Maharishi and the Vedic scholars at the Indian Institute of Maharishi's Vedic Science and Technology, who feel this transliteration produces the most accurate pronunciation of the original Sanskrit form.

Overview

My thesis, Physiological Effects of Transcendental Meditation: A Proposed Fourth Major State of Consciousness, was completed in 1970 in the Department of Physiology at the University of California at Los Angeles.

An excellent review of research on neuropeptides is given by Candace Pert (1986): The Wisdom of the Receptors: Neuropeptides, The Emotions and Bodymind, *Advances*, 3(3): 8–16.

A thorough understanding of the relationship between the unified field as described in the latest theories of modern science and the field of pure consciousness as described by Maharishi's Vedic Science is given in two brilliant articles by Dr. John Hagelin (1987): Is Consciousness the Unified Field? A Field Theorist's Perspective, *Modern Science and Vedic Science*, 1(1): 29–87, and (1989) Restructuring Physics from its Foundation in Light of Maharishi's Vedic Science, *Modern Science and Vedic Science*, 3(1): 3–72.

A brief introduction to Maharishi's Vedic Science and Technology is given by Dr. Kenneth Chandler (1987) in Modern Science and Vedic Science: An Introduction, *Modern Science and Vedic Science*, 1(1): 5–26.

The primary works of Maharishi Mahesh Yogi in which the basic principles and technologies of the Vedic paradigm are discussed are: *Science of Being and Art of Living: Transcendental Meditation* (New York: Signet, 1963); *On the Bhagavad-Gita: A Translation and Commentary, Chapters 1–6* (Baltimore:

Penguin/Arkana, 1967); *Life Supported by Natural Law* (Fairfield, IA: Maharishi International University Press, 1986); *Enlightenment to Every Individual and Invincibility to Every Nation* (Rheinweiler, W. Germany: Maharishi European Research University Press, 1978); *Maharishi Vedic University Inauguration* (Washington, DC: Age of Enlightenment Press, 1985); and *Maharishi's Absolute Theory of Government: Automation in Administration* (1992). Maharishi's discovery of the Constitution of the Universe is discussed more fully in Chapters 12 and 14; for references, see notes for those chapters.

Chapter 1

Dr. Orme-Johnson's views (1988) on the state of modern psychology, as well as an introduction to Maharishi's Vedic Psychology, are given The Cosmic Psyche—An Introduction to Maharishi's Vedic Psychology: The Fulfillment of Modern Psychology, *Modern Science and Vedic Science*, 2(2): 113–163.

Maharishi International University is accredited through the Ph.D. level, with 6 doctoral programs in physics, physiology, neuroscience of human consciousness, psychology, management, and the Science of Creative Intelligence; 10 master's programs in business admininistration, computer science, education, English, art, fine arts, higher education administration, mathematics, professional writing, and the Science of Creative Intelligence; and 14 undergraduate programs in physics, biology, psychology, mathematics, chemistry, computer science, electrical engineering, electro-mechanical engineering, electronics, business, government, literature, art, and the Science of Creative Intelligence.

A more complete understanding of the self-interacting dynamics of consciousness and the levels of the mind as explained by Maharishi is given in *Life Supported by Natural Law* and also in an article by Dr. Michael C. Dillbeck (1988), The Mechanics of Individual Intelligence Arising from the Field of Cosmic Intelligence—The Cosmic Psyche, *Modern Science and Vedic Science*, 2(3): 245–278.

A description of the Transcendental Meditation technique and higher states of consciousness is given in Maharishi's books *Science of Being and Art of Living: Transcendental Meditation* and *On the Bhagavad-Gita: A Translation and Commentary, Chapters 1–6*. Two other books that give a popular introduction to Transcendental Meditation are *Transcendental Meditation* by Robert Roth (New York: Donald I. Fine, 1987) and *The TM Book: How to Enjoy the Rest of Your Life* by Denise Denniston (Fairfield, IA: Fairfield Press, 1975).

Maurice Herzog's description of Annapurna appears in Herzofin, M.

Murphy, M., White, R. A., *The Psychic Side of Sports* (Redding, MA: Addison-Wesley, 1978, p. 30).

Chapter 2

Most of the original published research on the Transcendental Meditation and TM-Sidhi program is reprinted in *Scientific Research on Maharishi's Transcendental Meditation and TM-Sidhi Programme: Collected Papers*, Volumes 1–5. (Volume 1 is entitled *Scientific Research on the Transcendental Meditation Program*, and was published in 1977 in Rheinweiler, W. Germany, by Maharishi European Research University Press; Volumes 2–4 were published in Vlodrop, the Netherlands, by Maharishi Vedic University Press; and Volume 5 is in press in Fairfield, IA, at Maharishi International University Press.) Hereafter, these will be referred to as *Collected Papers*. In a previous book, *The Neurophysiology of Enlightenment* (Fairfield, IA: Maharishi International University Press, 1986), I have also given a thorough review of the research on the Transcendental Meditation and TM-Sidhi program. My original research includes several publications:

- Wallace, R. K. (1970), Physiological Effects of Transcendental Meditation, *Science, 167*: 1751–1754;
- Wallace, R. K., Benson, H., Wilson, A. F. (1971), A Wakeful Hypo-metabolic Physiologic State, *American Journal of Physiology, 221*(3): 795–799; and
- Wallace, R. K., Benson, H. (1972), The Physiology of Meditation, *Scientific American, 226*(2): 84–90.

The most recent review article is:

- Jevning, R., Wallace, R. K., Beldebach, M. (1992), The Physiology of Meditation: A Review. A Wakeful Hypometabolic Integrated Response, *Neuroscience, and Biobehavioral Reviews, 16*: 415–424.

Specific studies on respiratory changes during the Transcendental Meditation and TM-Sidhi program include:

- Allison, J. (1970), Respiratory Changes During Transcendental Meditation, *The Lancet, 1*(7651): 833–834;
- Farrow, J. T., Hebert, J. R. (1982), Breath Suspension During the Transcendental Meditation Technique, *Psychosomatic Medicine, 44*(2): 133–153;
- Wolkove, N., Kreisman, H., Darragh, D., Cohen, C., Frank, H. (1984), Effect of Transcendental Meditation on Breathing and Respiratory Control, *Journal of Applied Physiology: Respiratory, Environmental, and Exercise Physiology, 56*(3): 607–612; and

• Singh, B. (1984), Patients and Practitioners of Transcendental Meditation, *Psychosomatic Medicine, 4*: 347–362.

Studies on local metabolic changes include:

• Jevning, R., Wilson, A. F., O'Halloran, J. P., Walsh, R. N. (1983), Forearm Blood Flow and Metabolism During Stylized and Unstylized States of Decreased Activation, *American Journal of Physiology, 245, Regulatory, Integrative, and Comparative Physiology, 14*(1): R110–R116;

• Jevning, R., Wilson, A. F., Pirkle, H., O'Halloran, J. P., Walsh, R. N. (1983), Metabolic Control in a State of Decreased Activation: Modulation of Red Cell Metabolism, *American Journal of Physiology, 245: Cell Physiology, 14*: C457–C461;

• Jevning, R., Wilson, A. F., Smith, W. R., Morton, M. E. (1978), Redistribution of Blood Flow in Acute Hypometabolic Behavior, *American Journal of Physiology, 235*(4): R89–R92; and

• Wilson, A. F., Jevning, R., Guich, S. (1987), Marked Reduction of Forearm Carbon Dioxide Production During States of Decreased Metabolism, *Physiology and Behavior, 41*: 347–352.

References concerning changes in brain wave activity during TM include:

• Banquet, J. P. (1973), Spectral Analysis of the EEG in Meditation, *Electroencephalography and Clinical Neurophysiology, 35*: 143–151;

• Banquet, J. P., Sailhan, M. (1974), EEG Analysis of Spontaneous and Induced States of Consciousness, *Revue d'Electroencéphalographie et de Neurophysiologie Clinique, 4*: 445–453;

• Banquet, J. P., Sailhan, M. (1977), Quantified EEG Spectral Analysis of Sleep and Transcendental Meditation, Paper presented at the Second European Congress on Sleep Research, Rome, Italy, *Collected Papers*, Vol. 1; and

• Hebert, J. R., Lehmann, D. (1977), Theta Bursts: An EEG Pattern in Normal Subjects Practicing the Transcendental Meditation Technique, *Electroencephalography and Clinical Neurophysiology, 42*: 397–405.

References for the work on the measurement of EEG coherence and its use in studying astronauts include:

• Walter, D. O., Rhodes, J. M., Brown, D., Adey, W. R. (1966), Comprehensive Spectral Analysis of Human EEG Generators in Posterior Cerebral Regions, *Electroencephalography and Clinical Neurophysiology, 20*: 224–237;

• Walter, D. O., Kado, R. T., Rhodes, J. M., Adey, W. R. (1967), Electroencephalographic Baselines in Astronaut Candidates Estimated by Computation and Pattern Recognition Techniques, *Aerospace Medicine, 38*: 371–379; and

- Walter, D. O., Rhodes, J. M., Adey, W. R. (1967), Discriminating Among States of Consciousness by EEG Measurements: A Study of Four Subjects, *Electroencephalography and Clinical Neurophysiology, 22*: 22–29.

Studies on EEG power and coherence during Transcendental Meditation and the TM-Sidhi program include:

- Levine, P. H. (1976), The Coherence Spectral Array (COSPAR) and its Application to the Study of Spatial Ordering in the EEG, *Proceedings of the San Diego Bio-Medical Symposium, 15*: 237–247;
- Levine, P. H., Hebert, J. R., Haynes, C. T., Strobel, U. (1977), EEG Coherence during the Transcendental Meditation Technique, *Collected Papers*, Vol. 1;
- Badawi, K., Wallace, R. K., Orme-Johnson, D. W., Rouzeré, A. M. (1984), Electrophysiologic Characteristics of Respiratory Suspension Periods Occurring During the Practice of the Transcendental Meditation Program, *Psychosomatic Medicine, 46*(3): 267–276; and
- Dillbeck, M. C., Bronson, E. C. (1981), Short-Term Longitudinal Effects of the Transcendental Meditation Technique on EEG Power and Coherence, *International Journal of Neuroscience, 14*: 147–151.

Other important review articles on the Transcendental Meditation and TM-Sidhi program include:

- Dillbeck, M. C., Orme-Johnson, D. W. (1987), Physiological Differences Between Transcendental Meditation and Rest, *American Psychologist, 42*: 879–881;
- Orme-Johnson, D. W. (1973), Autonomic stability and Transcendental Meditation, *Psychosomatic Medicine, 35*: 341–349;
- Eppley, K. R., Abrams, A. I., Shear, J. (1989), Differential Effects of Relaxation Techniques on Trait Anxiety: A Meta-Analysis, *Journal of Clinical Psychology, 45*(6): 957–974; and
- Alexander, C. N., Rainforth, M. Y., Gelderloos, P. (1991), Transcendental Meditation, Self-Actualization, and Psychological Health: A Conceptual Overview and Statistical Meta-Analysis, *Journal of Social Behavior and Personality, 6*(5): 189–247.

A more complete description of higher states of consciousness is given by Maharishi in his books *Science of Being and Art of Living* and *On the Bhagavad-Gita*.

The passage from "Tintern Abbey" is quoted from Hayden, J. O. (Ed.), *William Wordsworth: The Poems* (Vol. I), (New Haven: Yale University Press, 1981, pp 358–359).

Chapter 3

An excellent account of the story of Guillemin's and Schally's research that led to the Nobel prize is given in a three-part series in *Science* magazine (1978) by Wade, N.: Guillemin and Schally: The Years in the Wilderness, *Science*, *200*: 279–282; Guillemin and Schally: The Three-Lap Race to Stockholm (ibid., pp. 411–415); and Guillemin and Schally: A Race Spurred by Rivalry (ibid., pp. 510–513).

Drs. Jevning and Wilson have published a number of articles on their biochemical research during the TM technique:

- Jevning, R., Pirkle, H. C., Wilson, A. F. (1977), Behavioral Alteration of Plasma Phenylalanine Concentration, *Physiology and Behavior*, *19*: 611–614;
- Jevning, R., Wilson, A. F., Davidson, J. M. (1978), Adrenocortical Activity During Meditation, *Hormones and Behavior*, *10*(1): 54–60;
- Jevning, R., Wilson, A. F., Vanderlaan, E. F. (1978), Plasma Prolactin and Growth Hormone During Meditation, *Psychosomatic Medicine*, *40*(4): 329–333; and
- O'Halloran, J. P., Jevning, R., Wilson, A. F., Skowsky, R., Walsh, R. N., Alexander, C. N. (1985), Hormonal Control in a State of Decreased Activation: Potentiation of Arginine Vasopressin Secretion, *Physiology and Behavior*, *35*: 591–595.

The reference for the long-term measurement of hormones in TM-Sidhi subjects is:

- Werner, O., Wallace, R. K., Charles, B., Janssen, G., Stryker, T., Chalmers, R. (1986), Long-Term Endocrinologic Changes in Subjects Practicing the Transcendental Meditation and TM-Sidhi Program, *Psychosomatic Medicine*, *48*(1–2): 59–66.

The references for Dr. Bujatti's and Dr. Walton's research on serotonin are:

- Bujatti, M., Riederer, P. (1976), Serotonin, Noradrenalin, Dopamine Metabolites in Transcendental Meditation Technique, *Journal of Neural Transmission*, *39*: 257–267;
- Walton, K. G., Lerom, M., Salerno, J., Wallace, R. K. (1981), Practice of the Transcendental Meditation (TM) and TM-Sidhi Program May Affect the Circadian Rhythm of Urinary 5-Hydroxyindole Excretion, *Society for Neuroscience Abstracts*, *7*: 48;
- MacLean, C. R. K., Walton, K. G., Wenneberg, S. R., Levitsky, D. K., Mandarino, J. V., Waziri, R., Schneider, R. H. (1992), Altered Cortisol Response to Stress after Four Months' Practice of the Transcendental Meditation Program, *Society for Neuroscience Abstracts*, *18*, 1541; and

• Walton, K. G., McCorkle, T., Hauser, T., Maclean, C., Wallace, R. K., Ieni, J., Meyerson, L. R. "Substance M," a Serotonin Modulator Candidate From Human Urine? In: Ehrlich, Y. H., Lenox, R. H., Kornecki, E., Berry, W.O. (Eds.), *Molecular Mechanisms of Neuronal Responsiveness*, Volume 221 of the series *Advances in Experimental Medicine and Biology* (New York: Plenum Press, 1987), 503–514.

Chapter 4

The studies on iatrogenic diseases are:

• Steel, K., Gertman, P. M., Crescenzi, C., Anderson, J. (March 12, 1981), Iatrogenic Illness on a General Medical Service at a University Hospital, *New England Journal of Medicine, 304*(11): 638–642; and
• Kramer, M. S., Hutchinson, T. A., Flegel, K. M., Naimark, L., Contardi, R., Leduc, D. G. (February 1985), Adverse Drug Reactions in General Pediatric Outpatients, *Journal of Pediatrics, 106*(2): 305–310.

The editorial, Need We Poison the Elderly So Often? is from *The Lancet*, 2(8601): 20–22, July 2, 1988.

One article on the excessive use of antibiotics is by Wang, J., Antibiotic Prophylaxis in Surgery, *Modern Medicine, 43*: 15, September 1, 1975.

The article on cancer is from Bailar, J., III, Smith, E. M. (May 8, 1986), Is There Progress Against Cancer? *New England Journal of Medicine, 314*(19): 1226–1232.

Articles and books on current problems in the treatment of heart disease include:

• Winslow, C. M., Kosecoff, J. B., Chassin, M., Kanouse, D. E., Brook, R. H. (Rand Corporation) (July 22/29, 1988), The Appropriateness of Performing Coronary Artery Bypass Surgery, *Journal of the American Medical Association, 260*(4): 505–509; and
• Ornish, D. et al. (1990), Can Lifestyle Changes Reverse Coronary Heart Disease? *The Lancet, 336*: 129–133.

A selection of studies on the effects of the TM and TM-Sidhi program on high blood pressure includes:

• Blackwell, B., Hanenson, I. B., Bloomfield, S. S., Magenheim, H. G., Nidich, S. I., Gartside, P. (1975), Effects of Transcendental Meditation on Blood Pressure: A Controlled Pilot Experiment, *Psychosomatic Medicine, 37*(1): 86;
• Simon, D. B., Oparil, S., Kimball, C. P. (1977), The Transcendental Meditation Program and Essential Hypertension, *Collected Papers*, Vol. 1;

- Agarwal, B. L., Kharbanda, A. Effect of Transcendental Meditation on Mild and Moderate Hypertension, *Collected Papers*, Vol. 3;
- Benson, H., Wallace, R. K. (1972), Decreased Blood Pressure in Hypertensive Subjects Who Practiced Meditation, *Supplement II* to *Circulation, 45 and 46*: 516; and
- Wallace, R. K., Silver, J., Mills, P., Dillbeck, M. C., Wagoner, D. E. (1983), Systolic Blood Pressure and Long-Term Practice of the Transcendental Meditation and TM-Sidhi Program: Effects of TM on Systolic Blood Pressure, *Psychosomatic Medicine, 45*(1): 41–46.

The most recent study on African Americans is reported in:

- Schneider, R., Alexander, C. N., Wallace, R. K. (1992), In Search of an Optimal Behavioral Treatment for Hypertension: A Review and Focus on Transcendental Meditation, in E. H. Johnson, W. D. Gentry, and S. Julius (Eds.), *Personality, Elevated Blood Pressure, and Essential Hypertension* (Washington, DC: Hemisphere Publishing), Chapter 14, pp. 291–316.

A selection of studies on the effects of the TM and TM-Sidhi program on cholesterol includes:

- Cooper, M. J., Aygen, M. M. (1979), A Relaxation Technique in the Management of Hypercholesterolemia, *Journal of Human Stress, 5*(4): 24–27; and
- Cooper, M. J., Aygen, M. M. (1978), Effect of Transcendental Meditation on Serum Cholesterol and Blood Pressure, *Harefuah, the Journal of the Israel Medical Association, 95*(1): 1–2.

A selection of studies on the effects of the TM and TM-Sidhi program on cardiovascular risk factors and other health problems includes:

- Benson, H., Wallace, R. K. (1972), Decreased Drug Abuse with Transcendental Meditation: A study of 1862 Subjects, in: Zarafonetis, C. J. D., (Ed.): *Drug Abuse: Proceedings of the International Conference* (Philadelphia: Lea and Febiger), pp. 369–376;
- Shafii, M., Lavely, R. A., Jaffe, R. D. Decrease in Cigarette Smoking Following Transcendental Meditation, *Collected Papers*, Vol. 3;
- Bauhofer, U. (1989), Das Programm der Transzendentalen Meditation in der Behandlung von Adipositas, *Collected Papers*, Vol. 3;
- Mills, P. J., Schneider, R. H., Hill, D., Walton, K. G., Wallace, R. K. (1990), Beta-Adrenergic Receptors and Sensitivity in Subjects Practicing Transcendental Meditation, *Journal of Psychosomatic Research, 34*(1): 29–33;
- Zamarra, J. W., Besseghini, I., Wittenberg, S. (1975), The Effects of the Transcendental Meditation Program on the Exercise Performance of Patients with Angina Pectoris, *Collected Papers*, Vol. 1; and
- Gelderloos, P., Walton, K. G., Orme-Johnson, D. W., Alexander, C. N. (1991), Effectiveness of the Transcendental Meditation Program in

Preventing and Treating Substance Misuse: A Review, *International Journal of the Addictions*, 26: 293–325.

The medical utilization studies are:

- Orme-Johnson, D.W. (1987), Medical Care Utilization and the Transcendental Meditation Program, *Psychosomatic Medicine*, *49*: 493–507; and
- Herron, R. F. (1992), The Impact of Transcendental Meditation Practice on Medical Expenditures, Doctoral Dissertation, Maharishi International University, Fairfield, IA.

Maharishi's book *Life Supported by Natural Law* includes an introduction to Maharishi Ayur-Ved.

Chapter 5

Please refer to the "General Note for All Chapters" on page 276 regarding pronunciation of Sanskrit terms.

The passages quoted from Maharishi regarding DNA, RNA, and the transition from consciousness to matter at the beginning of this chapter are from *Maharishi Vedic University Inauguration*. Maharishi's discussion of the tanmatras and mahabhutas is found in his translation and commentary on the Bhagavad-Gita, pp. 482–483.

Dr. Hagelin's two articles, from which his discussion of Panchamahabhuta theory in relation to modern physics is taken, are:

- Hagelin, J. S., (1987), Is Consciousness the Unified Field? A Field Theorist's Perspective, *Modern Science and Vedic Science 1*(1): 29–87; and
- Hagelin, J. S. (1989), Restructuring Physics from its Foundation in Light of Maharishi's Vedic Science, *Modern Science and Vedic Science 3*(1): 3–72. Dr. Hagelin's graphic is reprinted with slight modifications from the second article, where it originally appeared (p. 14).

Maharishi's comments about Dr. Triguna and pulse diagnosis are taken from *Maharishi Vedic University Inauguration*. He also discusses these topics in *Life Supported by Natural Law*.

Printed and videotaped materials are available from the College of Maharishi Ayur-Ved, Maharishi International University, Fairfield, IA 52557, which include a fuller explanation of body type and its relationship to diet, season and exercise, as well as a questionnaire designed to help the reader identify his or her own body type.

Reference information on immune function and digestion can be found in Horan, M. A., Fox, R. A. (1984), Aging and the Immune Response—A

Unifying Hypothesis? *Mechanisms of Aging and Development*, *26*: 165–181.
Previous work on body types by Western researchers includes:

- Smith, H. C. (1949), Psychometric Checks on Hypothesis Derived from Sheldon's Work on Physique and Temperament, *Journal of Personality*, *17*: 310–320; and
- Friedman, M., *Type A Behavior and Your Heart* (New York: Alfred A. Knopf, 1974).

Research on body types in Maharishi Ayur-Ved includes:

- Schneider, R. H., Wallace, R. K., Kasture, H. S., Averbach, R., Rothenberg, S., Robinson, D. K. (September 1985), Physiological and Psychological Correlates of Maharishi Ayur-Ved Psychosomatic Types, Paper presented at the Eighth World Congress of the International College of Psycho-somatic Medicine, Chicago, IL;
- Singh, R. H., Singh, N. B., Udupa, K. N. (1980), A Study of Tridosha as Neurohumors, *Journal of Research in Ayurveda and Siddha*, *1*(1): 1–20; and
- Udupa, K. N., *Stress and its Management by Yoga* (Delhi: Motilal, Banarsidas, 1985).

Studies on biological rhythms include:

- Halberg, F., Implications of Biologic Rhythms for Clinical Practice, in Krieger, D. T., Hughes, J. C. (Eds.), *Neuroendocrinology* (Sunderland, MA: Sinauer Associates, 1980, pp. 109–119); and
- Halberg, F., Haus, E., Cardoso, S. S., Schieving, L. E., Kuhl, J. F. W., Shiotsuka, R., Rosene, G., Pauly, J. E., Runge, W., Spalding, J. R., Lee, J. K., Good, R. A. (August 15, 1973), Toward a Chronotherapy of Neoplasia: Tolerance of Treatment Depends on Host Rhythms, *Experientia* (Basel), *29*: 909–934.

Chapter 6

Please refer to the "General Note for All Chapters" on page 276 regarding pronunciation of Sanskrit terms.

Maharishi's discussion of balance and imbalance mediated by the intellect is found in *Life Supported by Natural Law*. The quotations from Maharishi about Ved as the script of nature are from *Maharishi Vedic University Inauguration*. Materials from the College of Maharishi Ayur-Ved (see previous page) give a synopsis of the approaches of Maharishi Ayur-Ved.

The study on the effect of primordial sound on cancer cells is:

- Stephens, R. E., Sharma, H. M., Kauffman, E. M., Dudek, A. (1992), Effect of Different Sounds on Growth of Human Cancer Cell Lines in Vitro, *Federation Proceedings, 6*(5): A1934 (Abstract).

Dr. Susumu Ohno's work includes:

- Ohno, S. (1984), Repeats of Base Oligomers as the Primordial Coding Sequences of the Primeval Earth and Their Vestiges in Modern Genes, *Journal of Molecular Evolution, 20*(3–4): 313–321; and
- Ohno, S., Ohno, M. (1986), The All Pervasive Principle of Repetitious Recurrence Governs Not Only Coding Sequence Construction But Also Human Endeavor in Musical Composition, *Immunogenetics, 24*(2): 71–78.

The research on nasal cycles and EEG is reported in:

- Werntz, D. A., Bickford, R. G., Bloom, F. E., Shannahoff-Khalsa, D. S. (1983), Alternating Cerebral Hemispheric Activity and the Lateralization of Autonomic Nervous Function, *Human Neurobiology, 2*: 39–43.

Further discussion of left-right brain functioning is found in Gazzaniga, M. S., *The Bisected Brain* (New York: Appleton-Century-Crofts, 1970).

Other research on the approaches of Maharishi Ayur-Ved, particularly Maharishi Panchakarm purification procedures, includes:

- Schneider, R. H., Cavanaugh, K., Kasture, H. S., Rothenberg, S., Averbach, R., Robinson, D. K., Wallace, R.K. (1990), Health Promotion with a Traditional System of Natural Health Care: Maharishi Ayur-Veda, *Journal of Social Behavior and Personality, 5*(3): 1–27;
- Smith, D. E., Stevens, M. M. (1988), Pilot Project: The Effects of a Sesame Oil Mouth Rinse on the Number of Oral Bacteria Colony Types, Paper presented at the Third Annual Scientific Meeting of the College of Health Professions, Wichita State University;
- Stevens, M. M., Campbell, J., Smith, D. E., How, M. V., Benton, S. H., Bompurs, P. (June 1989), The Effects of a Sesame Oil Mouthrinse on the Number of Oral Bacteria Colony Types, Paper presented at the Cleveland International Symposium on Dental Hygiene, Ottawa, Canada;
- Salerno, J. M., Smith, D. E. (1991), The Use of Sesame Oil and Other Vegetable Oils in the Inhibition of Human Colon Cancer Cells in Vitro, *Anticancer Research, 11*: 209–216;
- Smith, D. E., Salerno, J. M. (1992), Selective Growth Inhibition of Human Malignant Melanoma Cell Line by Sesame Oil in Vitro, *Prostaglandins, Leukotrienes, and Essential Fatty Acids, 46*: 145–150;
- Bauhofer, U. et al (1988), Application of Maharishi Ayur-Ved in Infection with the Human Immune Deficiency Virus (HIV)—Case Reports, Pre-

sented at the Fourth International Conference on AIDS, Stockholm, Sweden; and

- Waldschütz, R. (1988), Physiological and Psychological Changes Associated with Ayurvedic Purification Treatment, *Erfahrungsheilkunde—Acta Medica Empirica—Zeitschrift für die ärztliche Praxis*, 2: 720–729.
- Sharma, H. M., Nidich, S. I., Sands, D., Smith, D. E. (in press), Improvement in Cardiovascular Risk Factors through Maharishi Panchakarma Purification Procedures, *Federation Proceedings*.

Chapter 7

The studies on Maharishi Ayur-Ved Bhasma Rasayana are:

- Nader, T., Neuberne, P., Schneider, G., Wurzner, P. (June 1987), Maharishi Ayurveda Bhasma Rasayana: Its Safety and Effectiveness in Animal Models of Diet-Induced Tissue Damage in Surgically Induced Brain Lesions and in Chemically Induced Cancer Lesions, Paper presented at the Twenty-Eighth Annual Meeting of the Society for Economic Botany, University of Illinois, Chicago, IL; and
- Nader, T., Buehe, D., Neuberne, P. (March 1987), Ayur-Vedic Rasayana Protects Against Kidney and Liver Damage in Rats Fed a Low-Lipotrope, High-Fat Diet, *Federation Proceedings*, 46(3): 959, Abstract 3747.

Dr. Hari Sharma's book is *Freedom from Disease: How to control Free Radicals, a major cause of aging and disease, A Scientist Rediscovers Prevention Oriented Natural Health Care: Maharishi Ayur-Ved* (Toronto: Veda Publishing, 1993).

Studies on Maharishi Amrit Kalash (MAK) include:

Research on MAK and Cancer

- Patel, V. K, Wang, J., Shen, R. N., Sharma, H. M. (1990), Reduction of Metastases of Lewis Lung Carcinoma by an Ayurvedic Food Supplement in Mice, *Nutrition Research*, 12: 51–61;
- Sharma, H. M., Dwivedi, C., Satter, B. C., Gudehithlu, K. P., Abou-issa, H., Malarkey, W., Tejawani, G. A. (1990), Antineoplastic Properties of Maharishi-4 Against DMBA-Induced Mammary Tumors in Rats, *Pharmacology, Biochemistry and Behavior*, 35: 767–773;
- Sharma, H. M., Krieger, J., Dwivedi, C. (1990), Antineoplastic Properties of Dietary Maharishi-4 and Maharishi Amrit Kalash Ayurvedic Food Supplements, *European Journal of Pharmacology*, 183: 193;
- Sharma, H. M., Satter, B., Dwivedi, C. (1988), Anticarcinogenic Activity of an Ayurvedic Food Supplement, *Proceedings of the 1988 Conference of the American Physiological Society/American Society of Pharmacology and Experimen-*

tal Therapeutics: Abstracts 86.1 and 86.2, A121;

- Prasad, K. N, Edwards-Prasad, J., Kenrotti, S., Brodie, C., Vernadakis, A. (1992), Ayurvedic (Science of Life) Agents Induce Differentiation in Murine Neuroblastoma Cells in Culture, *Neuropharmacology, 31*(6): 599–607;

- Johnston, B. H., Mirsalis, J., Hamilton, C. (1991), Chemotherapeutic Effects of an Ayurvedic Herbal Supplement on Mouse Papilloma, *The Pharmacologist, 3*: 39; and

- Wallace, R. K. (June 1987), Maharishi Amrit Kalash and Its Effect on Natural Killer Cells, Paper presented at the Twenty-Eighth Annual Meeting of the Society for Economic Botany, University of Illinois, Chicago.

MAK and the Immune System

- Dileepan, K. N., Patel, V., Sharma, H. M., Stechschulte, D. J. (1990), Priming of Splenic Lymphocytes After Ingestion of an Ayurvedic Herbal Food Supplement: Evidence for an Immunomodulatory Effect, *Biochemical Archives, 6*: 267–274;

- Patel, V., Dileepan, K. N., Stechschulte, D. J., Sharma, H. (March 20, 1988), Enhancement of Lymphoproliferative Responses by Maharishi Amrit Kalash (MAK) in Rats, *Federation Proceedings, 2*(5), Abstract no. 4740; and

- Glaser, J. L., Robinson, D. K., Wallace, R. K. (1988), Effect of Maharishi Amrit Kalash on Allergies, described in Maharishi Ayurveda: An Introduction to Recent Research, *Modern Science and Vedic Science, 2*(1): 89–108.

MAK and the Cardiovascular System

- Sharma, H. M., Feng, Y., Panganamala, R. V. (1989), Maharishi Amrit Kalash (MAK) Prevents Human Platelet Aggregation, *Clinica & Terapia Cardiovascolare, 8*(3): 227–230.

MAK and Psychophysiological Well-Being

- Sharma, H. M., Hanissian, S., Rattan, A. K., Stern, S. L., Tejwani, G. (January-March 1991), Effect of Maharishi Amrit Kalash on Brain Opioid Receptors and Neuropeptides, *Journal of Research and Education in Indian Medicine 10*(1): 1–8; and

- Hauser, T., Walton, K. G., Glaser, J., Wallace, R. K. (November 14, 1988), Naturally Occurring Ligand Inhibits Binding of [3H]-Imipramine to High Affinity Receptors, Paper presented at the 18th Annual Meeting of the Society for Neuroscience, Toronto, Ontario, Canada, Abstract 99.19.

MAK and Free Radicals

- Niwa, Y. (1991), Effect of Maharishi 4 and Maharishi 5 on Inflammatory Mediators—With Special Reference to Their Free Radical Scavenging Effect, *Indian Journal of Clinical Practice, 1*(8): 23–27;

- Dwivedi, C., Sharma, H. M., Dobrowski, S., Engineer, F. N. (1991), Inhibitory Effects of Maharishi-4 and Maharishi-5 on Microsomal Lipid Peroxidation, *Pharmacology, Biochemistry and Behavior, 39*: 649–652;
- Sharma, H. M., Hanna, A. N., Kauffman, E. M., Newman, H. A. (October 6–11, 1991), Inhibition in Vitro of Human LDL Oxidation by Maharishi Amrit Kalash (M-4 & M-5), Maharishi Coffee Substitute (MCS) and Men's Rasayana (MR), Paper presented at the International Atherosclerosis Society, 9th International Symposium on Atherosclerosis, Rosemont, IL, Abstract 112;
- Bondy, S., Hernandez, T. M., Mattia, C. (in press), Anti-Oxidant Properties of Two Herbal Preparations, *Biochemical Archives*; and
- Panganamala, R. V., Sharma, H. M. (October 6–11, 1991), Antioxidant and Antiplatelet Properties of Maharishi Amrit Kalash (M-4) in Hyper-cholesterolemic Rabbits, Paper presented at the International Atherosclerosis Society, 9th International Symposium on Atherosclerosis, Rosemont, IL, Abstracts 110 and 111.

In this and subsequent sections describing free radicals and Dr. Sharma's and Dr. Niwa's research on Maharishi Amrit Kalash as a free radical scavenger, I have drawn on a lecture Dr. Sharma gave at a conference at Maharishi International University, October 24, 1989. An article reporting on that lecture from the November 1989 issue of *The Source*, written by Roger Pelizzari, has been very helpful.

MAK and General Health

- Glaser, J. L. (1988), ibid.; and
- Gelderloos, P., Ahlström, H. H. B., Orme-Johnson, D. W., Robinson, D. K., Glaser, J. L., Wallace, R. K. (1990), Influence of Ayur-Vedic Herbal Preparation on Age Related Visual Discrimination, *International Journal of Psychosomatics, 37*(1–4): 25–29;

The National Cancer Institute studies are described by Barnard Sherman in "From Cancer Prevention to Life Extension: Research on Maharishi Amrit Kalash Proliferates," in the August 1991 issue of *MIU World*, p. 25.

A major study on the effects of aspirin is reported in The Steering Committee of the Physicians' Health Study Research Group—Preliminary Report (1988), Findings from the Aspirin Component of the Ongoing Physicians' Health Study, *New England Journal of Medicine, 318*(4): 262–264.

Chapter 8

The text of Maharishi's lecture on immortality appears in *Maharishi Mahesh Yogi, Thirty Years Around the World: Dawn of the Age of Enlightenment,*

Vol. 1, 1957–1964 (the Netherlands: Maharishi Vedic University Press, 1986, pp. 574–576).

Dr. Strehler's comments on immortality appear in Rosenfield, A., *Prolongevity* (Avon, 1983), which also reviews theories of aging.

There are many other books and articles that review various theories of aging, such as:

- Hayflick and Finch, (Eds.), *The Handbook of Aging* (New York: Van Nostrand Reinhold, 1977);
- Schneider, E. L., Rowe, J. W., *Handbook of the Biology of Aging*, 3rd Edition (San Diego: Academic Press, 1990).
- Walford, R., *Maximum Life Span* (New York: Norton, 1983);
- Sacher, G. A. (April, 1978), Longevity, Aging, and Death: An Evolutionary Perspective, *The Gerontologist, 18*(2): 112–119; and
- Rosenfeld, A., *Prolongevity II: An Updated Report on the Scientific Prospects for Adding Good Years to Life* (New York: H. Holt, 1987).

Dr. Cutler's remarks are quoted in an interview in the October 1986 issue of *Omni* (Weintraub, P., *9*(1): 108–114, 174–181).

The warning on the potential side effects of life-extension programs is quoted from Schneider, E. L., Reed, J. D., Jr. (1985), Life Extension, *New England Journal of Medicine, 312*(18): 1159–1168.

Longevity factors are discussed in Palmore, E. (Ed.), *Normal Aging II, Reports from the Duke Longitudinal Study*, 1970–1973 (Durham, NC: Duke University Press, 1974).

Research on the Transcendental Meditation and TM-Sidhi program and aging includes:

- Wallace, R. K., Dillbeck, M. C., Jacobe, E., Harrington, B. (1982), The Effects of the Transcendental Meditation and TM-Sidhi Program on the Aging Process, *International Journal of Neuroscience, 16*: 53–58;
- Toomey, M., Pennington, B., Chalmers, R., Clements, G. (1989), The Practice of the Transcendental Meditation and TM-Sidhi Program Reverses the Physiological Aging Process, *Collected Papers*, Vol. 3;
- Toomey, M., Chalmers, R., Clements, G. (1989), The Transcendental Meditation and TM-Sidhi Programme Reverses the Physiological Ageing Process: A Longitudinal Study, *Collected Papers*, Vol. 3;
- Glaser, J. L., Brind, J. L., Vogelman, J. H. Eisner, M. J., Dillbeck, M. C. Wallace, R. K., Chopra, D, Orentreich, N. (1986), Elevated Serum Dehydroepiandrosterone Sulfate Levels in Practitioners of the Transcendental Meditation (TM) and TM-Sidhi Program, *Journal of Behavioral Medicine, 15*(4): 327–334;
- Alexander, C. N., Chandler, H. M., Langer, E. J., Davies, J. L., Newman, R.

I. (1989), Transcendental Meditation, Mindfulness and Longevity—An Experimental Study with the Elderly, *Journal of Personality and Social Psychology*, 57(6): 950–964;

- Goddard, P. H. (1989), Reduced Age Related Declines of P300 Latency in Elderly Practicing Transcendental Meditation, *Psychophysiology*, 26: 529; and
- Miishov, S. (1992), Endogenous Evoked Potentials in Subjects Practicing Transcendental Meditation, Doctoral Dissertation, Department of Clinical Neurophysiology, Zagreb University.

An excellent summary of Maharishi's views on immortality, from which the passages from him are quoted, is given in *Science, Consciousness and Ageing: Proceedings of the International Conference* (January 19–20, 1980), Rheinweiler, W. Germany: Maharishi European University Press.

Chapter 9

An excellent review article on the Maharishi Effect is Orme-Johnson, D. W., Dillbeck, M. C. (1987), Maharishi's Program to Create World Peace: Theory and Research, *Modern Science and Vedic Science*, 1(2): 207–259. A more popular review is given in a book by Robert Oates, *Creating Heaven on Earth* (Fairfield, IA: Heaven on Earth Publications, 1990).

Original studies on the Maharishi Effect include:

- Borland, C., Landrith III, G. (1977), Improved Quality of City Life Through the Transcendental Meditation Program: Decreased Crime Rate, *Collected Papers*, Vol.1;
- Dillbeck, M. C., Landrith III, G., Orme-Johnson, D. W. (1981), The Transcendental Meditation Program and Crime Rate Change in a Sample of Forty-Eight Cities, *Journal of Crime and Justice*, 4: 25–45; and
- Dillbeck, M. C., Banus, C. B., Polanzi, C., Landrith III, G. S. (1988), Test of a Field Model of Consciousness and Social Change: The Transcendental Meditation and TM-Sidhi Program and Decreased Urban Crime, *The Journal of Mind and Behavior*, 9(4): 457–486.

Studies up to 1978 on the Extended Maharishi Effect include:

- Orme-Johnson, D. W., Dillbeck, M. C., Bousquet, J. G., Alexander, C. N. (1990), The World Peace Project of 1978: An Experimental Analysis of Achieving World Peace through the Maharishi Technology of the Unified Field, *Collected Papers*, Vol. 4.

Also, *The Maharishi Effect: Creating Coherence in World Consciousness, Promoting Positive and Evolutionary Trends throughout the World* (Fairfield, IA: MIU Press, 1990) contains a detailed review of 38 studies on the Maharishi

Effect—at the level of cities, states, nations, conflicts between nations, and the entire world. (See also notes for Chapter 11.)

Sections of Jon Levy's guest editorial, "Technology of Consciousness Could Foster World Peace," from the December 7, 1978 issue of the *Ithaca Journal*, are reprinted with permission from the author.

Chapter 10

A full description of the Yogic Flying news events and complete texts of press conference participants' speeches and news reports (both from the first competition in Washington, D.C., and from subsequent such events in 1986 around the world) can be found in: *Maharishi's Programme to Create World Peace: Global Inauguration* (Washington, DC: Age of Enlightenment Press, 1987). The news report by Alex Van Oss about the "Yogic Flying Competition by Meditators" was originally broadcast on National Public Radio's "All Things Considered" on July 11, 1986, and is used with the permission of National Public Radio. © 1986 by National Public Radio.®

Research on Yogic Flying includes:

- Orme-Johnson, D. W., Gelderloos, P. (1988), Topographic EEG Brain Mapping During "Yogic Flying," *International Journal of Neuroscience, 38*: 427–434; and
- Travis, F. T., Orme-Johnson, D. W. (1990), EEG Coherence and Power During Yogic Flying, *International Journal of Neuroscience, 54*: 1–12.

The theories of quantum effects in the brain are described in Domash, L. H. (1975), The Transcendental Meditation Technique and Quantum Physics: Is Pure Consciousness a Macroscopic Quantum State in the Brain? *Collected Papers*, Vol. 1. A more complete presentation of Dr. Hagelin's discussion of Maharishi's field model of consciousness appears in his two articles referenced in Chapter 5.

Application of these principles to health and theories of brain functioning is discussed in:

- Dr. Deepak Chopra's book *Quantum Healing* (New York: Bantam, 1989);
- Dr. Chopra's article (1987), Bliss and the Quantum Mechanical Body, *Modern Science and Vedic Science, 2*: 61–74; as well as
- Eccles, J. C., (1986), Do Mental Events Cause Neural Events Analogously to the Probability Fields of Quantum Mechanics? *Proceedings of the Royal Society of London, B 227*: 411–428.

Maharishi discusses the TM-Sidhi program and the Maharishi Effect in several publications, including *Life Supported by Natural Law*, *Enlightenment and Invincibility*, and *Maharishi's Programme to Create World Peace: Global Inauguration*, from which the passages from Maharishi are quoted. In addition, an excellent review of the theory and research on Maharishi's TM-Sidhi program and Yogic Flying is found in:

- Gelderloos, P., Berg, W. P. van den (1989), Maharishi's TM-Sidhi Program: Participating in the Infinite Creativity of Nature to Enliven the Totality of the Cosmic Psyche in All Aspects of Life, *Modern Science and Vedic Science 2*(4), 374–412.

The Secret of the Golden Flower, A Chinese Book of Life is translated by Richard Wilhelm (London: Kegan Paul, Trench, Trubner, 1962). St. Theresa's description of rapture is quoted from *St. Teresa of Avila* by Stephen Clissold (London: Sheldon Press, 1982). *The Origins of Culture* is by Sir Edward Burnett Tylor (New York: Harper & Row, 1958). *Butler's Lives of the Saints, Complete Edition* is revised and supplemented by Herbert Thurston, S.J., and Donald Attwater (New York: P. J. Kennedy and Sons, 1962).

Maharishi's comments on the application of Yog in Yogic Flying appear in *Maharishi's Programme to Create World Peace: Global Inauguration* (p. vii). His comments from his 1986 lecture on the evolutionary nature of the unified field promoted through the TM-Sidhi program are also found in that book.

Chapter 11

As noted in the references for Chapter 9, a survey of 38 studies on the Maharishi Effect is found in *The Maharishi Effect*. This research includes:

- Orme-Johnson, D. W., Alexander, C. N., Davies, J. L., Chandler, H. M., Larimore, W. E. (1988), International Peace Project in the Middle East: The Effects of the Maharishi Technology of the Unified Field, *Journal of Conflict Resolution, 32*: 776–812;
- Orme-Johnson, D. W., Cavanaugh, K. L., Alexander, C. N., Gelderloos, P., Dillbeck, M. C., Lanford, A. G., Nader, T. A. (1991), The Influence of the Maharishi Technology of the Unified Field on World Events and Global Social Indicators: The Effects of the Taste of Utopia Assembly, *Collected Papers*, Vol. 4;
- Davies, J. L. (1988), Alleviating Political Violence through Enhancing Coherence in Collective Consciousness: Impact Assessment Analysis of the Lebanon War, *Dissertation Abstracts International, 49*(8): 2381A;
- Dillbeck, M. C., Cavanaugh, K. L., Glenn, T., Orme-Johnson, D. W., Mittlefehldt, V. (1987), Consciousness as a Field: The Transcendental

Meditation and TM-Sidhi Program and Changes in Social Indicators, *The Journal of Mind and Behavior,* 8(1): 67–104;

- Orme-Johnson, D. W., Dillbeck, M. C. (1991), Results of the World Peace Assembly on Vedic Science Held in Washington, D.C., *Collected Papers,* Vol. 4;
- Orme-Johnson, D. W., Gelderloos, P., Dillbeck, M. C. (1988), The Effects of the Maharishi Technology of the Unified Field on the U.S. Quality of Life (1960–1984), *Social Science Perspectives Journal,* 2: 127–146;
- Reeks, D. (1990), Improved Quality of Life in Iowa through the Maharishi Effect, *Dissertation Abstracts International,* 51(12): 6155B; and
- Cavanaugh, K. L., King, K. D., Ertuna, C. (1989), A Multiple-Input Transfer Function Model of Okun's Misery Index: An Empirical Test of the Maharishi Effect, Paper presented at the Annual Meeting of the American Statistical Association, Washington, D.C., August 6–10, 1989. (An abridged version of this paper appeared in *Proceedings of the American Statistical Association, Business and Economics Statistics Section,* Alexandria, VA: American Statistical Association.)

The research on U.S.-Soviet relations is:

- Gelderloos, P., Frid, J. F., Goddard, P. H., Xue, X., Loliger, S. (1988), Creating World Peace through the Collective Practice of the Maharishi Technology of the Unified Field: Improved U.S.-Soviet Relations, *Social Science Perspectives Journal,* 2(4): 80–94

Chapter 12

The announcements of Maharishi's offers to governments appeared in major newspapers and magazines throughout the world in 1990 and 1991, including *The Washington Post,* the *Wall Street Journal,* the *International Herald Tribune, The Times* (London), and the *Hindustan Times* (New Delhi). The principle that governments are only an innocent mirror of collective consciousness has been expressed by Maharishi in a number of his publications, including *Enlightenment and Invincibility, Life Supported by Natural Law, and Maharishi's Absolute Theory of Government.*

The Constitution of the Universe was first described at length by Maharishi in a global telecast via satellite on January 12, 1991. Maharishi's Master Plan to Create Heaven on Earth is summarized in a 1,500-page book of the same title (Vlodrop, the Netherlands: Maharishi Vedic University Press, in press). An overview of this document is given in *Maharishi's Master Plan to Create Heaven on Earth* (Vlodrop, the Netherlands: Maharishi Vedic University Press, 1991).

Chapter 13

Please refer to the "General Note for All Chapters" on page 276 regarding pronunciation of Sanskrit terms.

Maharishi's initial statements on Ved and the mass of cells were made during a lecture in India in 1986; a similar discussion appears in the first edition (1974) of the Maharishi International University catalogue. Maharishi's definitions of his Vedic Science have appeared in "Maharishi's Vedic Science: Definition and Scope," in the *Manifesto* of the Natural Law Party, England, 1992. The discussion of the sequential unfoldment of natural law and the Vedic literature in Maharishi's Vedic Science is based on that found in several sources, including: *Maharishi's Absolute Theory of Government: Automation in Administration, Maharishi Vedic University Inauguration, Life Supported by Natural Law*, and Maharishi Vedic University *Bulletin* (1985). The diagram on page 227 is reprinted with slight modifications from the original, which appears in *Life Supported by Natural Law*. The diagram on page 229 is reprinted from the original in *Maharishi's Absolute Theory of Government*.

An excellent discussion of the unfoldment of Vedic literature in Maharishi's Vedic Science is given by Dr. Michael C. Dillbeck (1988) in The Mechanics of Individual Intelligence Arising from the Field of Cosmic Intelligence—The Cosmic Psyche, *Modern Science and Vedic Science*, 2(3): 245–278. Maharishi's concluding statements about Maharishi Ayur-Ved, pulse diagnosis, and the Vedic literature were made during a lecture in December 1992 in Vlodrop, the Netherlands.

Chapter 14

Please refer to the "General Note for All Chapters" on page 276 regarding pronunciation of Sanskrit terms.

The graphics showing the first verses of Rik Ved and the Lagrangian of the superstring are reprinted from the full-page announcement of the Constitution of the Universe entitled "Modern Science and Ancient Vedic Science Reveal the Constitution of the Universe: The Source of All Order and Harmony Displayed throughout the Universe, Discovered through Maharishi's Vedic Science, Verified by Modern Science." That announcement appeared in the international press throughout the world in January 1992, including the Toronto *Globe and Mail*, the Ottawa *Citizen*, the *International Herald Tribune, The Financial Times* (Great Britain and International), the *Wall Street Journal* (Europe, Asia, and U.S.), and *The Washington Post*. The same announcement is also a source for the discussion of Maharishi's Apaurusheya Bhashya of the Ved. Other primary sources include: *Maharishi's Absolute*

Theory of Government: Automation in Administration, Maharishi Vedic University Inauguration, an address by Maharishi to a press conference in Washington, D.C., held by the Natural Law Party of the United States on June 25, 1992, and Dr. Michael Dillbeck's article in *Modern Science and Vedic Science* which was referenced in Chapter 13. The diagrams on pages 239 and 243 are reprinted (the second with slight modifications) from Dr. Dillbeck's article.

Maharishi's description of the collapse of infinity to a point was presented in a lecture in January 1991 in Maastricht, the Netherlands. The discussions of silence and dynamism, support of nature, administration through natural law, and *Yatinam Brahma bhavati sarathih* are more fully elaborated in *Maharishi's Absolute Theory of Government.* Maharishi's quoted statements on are these subjects taken from these sources.

Chapter 15

Maharishi's discussion of DNA is from a lecture in India in 1986, *Maharishi Vedic University Inauguration* and *Maharishi's Absolute Theory of Government.*

The discussion and chart on DNA and the Brahmanas are based on those in Wallace, R. K., Fagan, J., Pasco, D. (1988), Vedic Physiology, *Modern Science and Vedic Science 2*: 2–59. The correspondences between DNA and the Richo Akshare verse of Rik Ved have been developed as part of a series of curriculum materials and charts that include many other academic disciplines and professions. These have been prepared by the faculty of Maharishi International University and Maharishi Vedic University Press for use in Maharishi Vedic Universities around the world.

Chapter 16

The research on experience and the brain includes:

- Rosenzweig, M. R., Bennett, E. L., Diamond, M. C. (1972), Brain Changes in Response to Experience, *Scientific American, 226*: 22–29; and
- Diamond, C., Ingham, C. A., Johnson, R. E., Bennett, E. L., Rosenzweig, M. R. (1976), Effects of Environment on Morphology of Rat Cerebral Cortex and Hippocampus, *Journal of Neurobiology, 1*: 75–86.

Maharishi's comments on the loss and revival of knowledge are greatly elaborated in the preface to his book *On the Bhagavad-Gita: A Translation and Commentary, Chapters 1–6,* p. 16.

Other points of Maharishi's discussion are taken from Maharishi's commentary on the Bhagavad-Gita, noted above; *Maharishi Mahesh Yogi, Thirty*

Years Around the World: Dawn of the Age of Enlightenment, Vol. 1, 1957–1964; *Maharishi Vedic University Inauguration*, and Maharishi's introductory statements in the journal *Modern Science and Vedic Science*, pp. i–ii.

Index

A

'*A*', 238, 240

abhyang, 107

absolute, 79, 135, 155, 173, 201, 230, 249

academic performance, 42

acetylcholine, 82, 269

ACTH, 46

acupuncture, 132–133

Adey, Ross, 39

administration of nature, 253

administration through natural law, 203–205

adrenaline, 4, 52, 57

Age of Enlightenment, 189

aging, 41, 58, 63, 85, 87, 113, 116, 120, 128–130, 135–147

aging genes, 138

agni, 71, 73, 75, 80

agnis, 86

Aham Brahmasmi, 273

Ahamkar, 241

Ak, 237–238, 240

akash, 71–73, 75, 80, 241

Alexander, Charles, 41, 184

alcohol consumption, 120, 142, 188–189

Alliance with Nature's Government, 195–197

ama, 87

amino acids, 49, 254

anatomy of consciousness, 18, 22, 26, 29, 42, 70

angina pectoris, 62

antidiuretic hormone, 49

antioxidants, 123, 139

anxiety, 41, 80, 106, 143, 162, 195, 204

anyonyabhav, 238–239

Apaurusheya, 218, 235

Apaurusheya Bhashya of the Ved, Maharishi's, 235–236 240, 242, 244, 253

Aranyakas, 221–222, 225, 257–259

Armenia, TM program in, 192–193

Arnold, Julia T., 118

Aroma therapy, 102–103

arthritis, 80, 120, 125, 140

asanas, 88

asthma, 81

Atharv Ved, 217, 221–222, 224–225, 227

atherosclerosis, 120, 124–125, 130

athletes, 80, 88–89

atyantabhav, 238–239

avyakt, 70, 242

awareness,

comprehending the interaction between silence and dynamism, 245;

change of during illness, 93;

different states of, 36;

during witnessing, 27;

expression of the lively field of all the laws of nature, 250;

fine fabrics of the, 271

having the Constitution of the Universe fully lively in the, 247;

how to expand, 12;

in higher states of consciousness, 29;

in *pragyaparadh,* 95;

in the state of enlightenment, 146–147;

limited, 10;

of the *vaidya* 77–79;

permanent establishment of pure consciousness in cosmic consciousness, 38–41;

of the great enlightened sages, 218–219;

opening itself to the field of all possibilities, 220–221;

pure, 19–21, 33, 218;

simplest state of, 180; 215, 207, 209, 233, 246, 273;

unbounded, 47, 60;